THE RELATIONSHIP BEWTEEN PREDNISONE USE, SELF-ESTEEM, SOCIAL INTIMACY AND ILLNESS INTRUSION

A dissertation submitted to the faculty of

the California School of Professional Psychology

in partial fulfillment of the requirements for the degree of

Doctor of Philosophy at

Alliant International University, Los Angeles, California

by

Kristin Plachetka Katz M.A.

April 14, 2009

UMI Number: 3368137

Copyright 2009 by
Katz, Kristin Plachetka

INFORMATION TO USERS

The quality of this reproduction is dependent upon the quality of the copy submitted. Broken or indistinct print, colored or poor quality illustrations and photographs, print bleed-through, substandard margins, and improper alignment can adversely affect reproduction.
In the unlikely event that the author did not send a complete manuscript and there are missing pages, these will be noted. Also, if unauthorized copyright material had to be removed, a note will indicate the deletion.

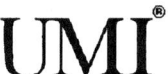

UMI Microform 3368137
Copyright 2009 by ProQuest LLC
All rights reserved. This microform edition is protected against unauthorized copying under Title 17, United States Code.

ProQuest LLC
789 East Eisenhower Parkway
P.O. Box 1346
Ann Arbor, MI 48106-1346

Copyright by
Kristin Plachetka Katz
2009

ALLIANT INTERNATION UNIVERSITY Los Angeles

The dissertation of Kristin Plachetka Katz, directed and approved
By the candidate's Committee, has been accepted by the
Faculty of the California School of Professional Psychology
in partial fulfillment of the requirement for the Degree of

DOCTOR OF PHILOSPHY

March 17, 2009
Date

Dissertation Committee:

Tracy Heller, Ph.D., Chairperson

Terece Bell, Ph.D.

Nick Noviello, Ph.D.

TABLE OF CONTENTS

List of Tables..iv
List of Appendices......................................v
Acknowledgments..vi
Vita..vii
Abstract of Dissertation..............................viii

CHAPTER 1   INTRODUCTION..........................1
    Statement of Purpose................................4
    Importance of the Study.............................5

CHAPTER II   REVIEW OF THE LITERATURE.................6
    Self-Esteem and Coping with Chronic Illness.........6
    Long Term Effect of Chronic Illness and Self-Esteem..12
    Self-Image and Chronic Illness.....................14
    Self-Esteem and Autonomy...........................15
    Chronic Illness and Social Support.................16
    Intimate Relationships and Social Support..........25
    Illness Intrusiveness..............................30
    The Effects of Steroid Use.........................31
    Perceived Medication Side Effects..................33
    Side Effects of Psychological Medications..........37
    Affect and Medication..............................38
    Hypotheses...40
    Definition of Terms................................42

CHAPTER III   METHODS................................44
    Participants.......................................44
    Measures...47
    Demographics Questionnaire.........................47
        Rosenberg Self-Esteem Scale....................47
        Miller Social Intimacy Scale...................48
        Adapted Illness Intrusiveness Rating...........49
    Procedures...50
    Design...51

CHAPTER IV   RESULTS.................................52
    Demographic and Study Variables....................52
    Correlation of Study Variables.....................55

    Comparison of Prednisone Group and Control Group...................57
    Hypotheses..57
    Bonferroni Correction...65
    Post Hoc Analysis...66

CHAPTER V   DISSCUSSION..67
    Clinical Implications...71
    Assumptions and Limitations...72
    Further Research..73

REFERENCES..75
APPENDICES..81

LIST OF TABLES

Table 1 Descriptive Statistics of Demographic Variables..................................45

Table 2 Medical Information for Participants..53

Table 3 Correlation of Demographic and Study Variables.................................56

Table 4 Pearson's Correlation Matrix of Side Effects and Self-Esteem, Social Intimacy and Illness Intrusion for the Prednisone Group Only..59

Table 5 Pearson's Correlation Matrix of Side Effects and Self-Esteem, Social Intimacy and Illness Intrusion for the Prednisone and Control Group................................61

LIST OF APPENDICES

Appendix A Informed Consent Form……………………………………………..…..81

Appendix B Rosenberg Self-Esteem Scale……………………………………….……..83

Appendix C Miller Social Intimacy Scale………………………………………...........84

Appendix D Adapted Illness Intrusiveness Ratings……………………………….……85

Appendix E Demographics Questionnaire…………………………………….………..86

Acknowledgments

First I would like to thank my amazing committee, Dr. Tracy Heller, Dr. Terece Bell, and Dr. Nick Noviello, for all of their guidance and support throughout the dissertation process. I would especially like to acknowledge my dissertation chair, Dr. Heller, for all of her knowledge and encouragement. She was a wonderful mentor and helped me survive the hectic dissertation process.

I would like to thank my parents, Dorothy, Michael and Augie, for all of their love, support and encouragement through the long journey of graduate school and my entire academic career. They have always encouraged me to do my best and I would not have accomplished what I have if it weren't for them. And I would like to thank my sister Victoria, for always putting a smile on my face and distracting me from the stresses of graduate school.

Finally, I would like to thank my husband, Aron, who participated in many discussions about dissertation and never seem bored by the subject. He is so supportive in big and small ways and I could never thank him enough. Graduate school has been a long journey for us both, and it was made easier having him by my side.

VITA

Kristin M. Plachetka Katz

2004	--	B.A., University of San Francisco
2006-2007	--	Practicum Intern, AIDS Services Foundation of Orange County Irvine, California
2007	--	M.A., California School of Professional Psychology, Los Angeles
2007-2008	--	Intern, United American Indian Involvement, Seven Generations Child and Family Counseling Services Los Angeles, California
2008-Present	--	Intern, United American Indian Involvement, Robert Sundance Family Wellness Center Los Angeles, California

ABSTRACT OF THE DISSERTATION

The Relationship Between Prednisone Use,

Self-Esteem and Social Intimacy and Illness Intrusion

By

Kristin M. Plachetka Katz

Doctor of Philosophy

California School of Professional Psychology
Alliant International University Los Angeles
2009

Tracy Heller, Ph.D., Chairperson

    The current study investigated the relationship between self-esteem, social intimacy and illness intrusion in individuals with a chronic illness currently taking prednisone and individuals with a chronic illness not currently taking prednisone. The researcher hypothesized that participants with a chronic illness currently taking prednisone would have lower self-esteem, less satisfying social relationships and more illness intrusion than participants with a chronic illness who were not currently taking prednisone. It was also hypothesized that increased severity of side effects would be related to lower self-esteem, less satisfying social relationships and more illness intrusion in participants currently taking prednisone compared to participants not currently taking prednisone.

    One hundred and one participants were recruited from internet advertisements. There were 41 participants in the group currently taking prednisone and 60 participants in the group of participants with a chronic illness but not currently using prednisone. Participants were directed to a surveymonkey.com account. Participants reported demographic information, medical information, as well as completed the Rosenberg Self-Esteem Scale (1989), Miller Social Intimacy Scale (1982) and the Adapted Illness Intrusiveness Scale (2001).

    Results were not statistically significant for the relationship between participants currently using prednisone, self-esteem, social intimacy and illness intrusion. However, a significant relationship between specific side effects and self-esteem, social intimacy and illness intrusion was found for all participants currently taking medication, regardless of the medication being taken.

CHAPTER 1

INTRODUCTION

Chronic physical illness has been shown to impact one's self-concept, body image, quality of life, social functioning, and self-esteem (Bishop, 2005; Ireys, Gross, Werthamer-Larsson, Kolodner, 1994; Liveneh & Antonak, 2005; Meijer, Sinnema, Bijstra, Mellenbergh, & Wolters, 2000; Norton, Manne, Rubin, Hernandez, Carlson, Bergman, & Rosenblum, 2005; Walsh & Walsh, 2001). Furthermore, the medications used to treat chronic illnesses in and of themselves have potential side effects that may serve to exacerbate the impact of chronic illness on well-being, body image, and self-esteem (Carrick, Mitchell, Powell, & Lloyd, 2004; Fornari, Dancyger, La Monaca, Budman, Goodman, Kabo, & Katz, 2001; Martinez, Kemper, Diamond, & Wagner, 2005).

Many medications can result in various physical side effects and both the experience of having a chronic illness and the physical side effects that may result from treatment can impact one's self-esteem. A medication widely used in the treatment of chronic physical illness is prednisone. Prednisone was the sixteenth most prescribed medication in the United States in 2000, according to the World Almanac and Book of Facts (2003). Prednisone is used to treat a variety of inflammatory illnesses in children and adults. Prednisone can result in a variety of physical and emotional side effects that could have an impact on a person's self-esteem. Prednisone has a variety of side effects such as facial swelling, suppression of the immune system, facial and body hair growth, stretch marks, osteoporosis, mood swings, insomnia, thrush, acne, hair loss and weight gain (Kalibjian, 2003; Sklar, 2002). These types of side effects may have an effect on one's well-being, specifically self-esteem and social intimacy above and beyond the impact due to the chronic illness alone.

Self-esteem is central to the understanding and appreciation of oneself. Terms like self-esteem, self-worth, self-respect and self-acceptance can many times be used interchangeably (Abraido-Lanza, 2004; Conn, Taylor, & Hayes, 1992; Silver, Bauman, & Ireys, 1995). Self-esteem is conceptualized as positive or negative feelings about one's self (Silver et al., 1995). Self-esteem is thought of as respect and acceptance for oneself and may have an impact on affect (Silver et al., 1995). Self-esteem can have an impact on one's perception of self and psychological well-being.

Decreased physical activity due to illness and pain can have a long term negative effect on multiple aspects of life and well-being (van Lankveld, Naring, van't Pad Bosch, & van de Putte, 2000). Negative body image was associated with the presence of symptoms, either due to chronic illness or to medication side effects (Martinez, Kemper, Diamond, & Wagner, 2005). Negative body image could have an impact on self-esteem. Being chronically ill has an impact on a patient's independence which can directly affect self-esteem (Covino, Dirks, Kinsmans, & Seidel, 1982).

Social support is an interaction of social and emotional resources between the individual and his or her environment which can have an impact on psychological well-being (Suurmeijer, Reuvekamp, & Aldenkamp, 2001). Illness can restrict one's ability to access social relationships which can have an effect on social intimacy (Meijer, Sinnema, Bijstra, Mellenbergh, & Wolters, 2000). Chronic illness can have as much of an impact on one's social life as a physical condition (Gregory, 2005; Scherman, Dahlgren, & Lowhagen, 2002). Being unable to maintain a social life due to a chronic illness had a negative impact on quality of life and self-esteem (Nicolson & Anderson, 2003). Partners of people with chronic illnesses are affected and impacted by their partner's illness (Skerrett, 2003). Huurre and Aro (2002) found that adults with limiting chronic illness had lower self-esteem and were less likely to be married or living with someone, compared to healthy individuals and those whose chronic illness was not limiting. Self-esteem and social relationships can be greatly affected by chronic illness and medication use.

The way one views oneself could be dramatically impacted by medication physical side effects which could then lower one's self esteem. Although many of the side effects are temporary or reversible, the experience for the individual still may leave a lasting effect of decreased self-esteem. Although having a chronic illness can affect one's self-esteem, the physical side effects from prednisone may contribute to a more drastic change in image which produces a more dramatic effect on self-esteem. One's perception of oneself can also affect external relationships and intimacy with others. Conversely, intimacy and close interpersonal relationships have been shown to be a predictor of healthy psychological and physiological functioning (Miller & Lefcourt, 1982). Social resources are strongly related to quality of life in chronically ill women (Bloom, Stewart, Johnston, & Banks, 1998). Intimate relationships can positively affect the way one responds to stress (Miller & Lefcourt, 1982). Intimate relationships can help individuals cope with the stress of life changing situations. Participating in intimate relationships can help lessen the stress of being ill and taking medications daily.

Illness intrusiveness measures the way illness disrupts lifestyle, activities, well-being and quality of life. Illness intrusiveness refers to not only the interference of a disease but also the impact of treatment (Devins et al.,2001). The impact on illness intrusion is more distressing for younger individuals than older ones (Devins, Bezjak, Mah, Loblaw, & Gotowiec, 2006). Illness intrusion encompasses the impact of illness on physical well-being, work and finances, social, sexual and family relations. In this study, illness intrusion will be examined to investigate the impact due to prednisone use, beyond that of having a chronic illness. This study proposes that prednisone use may be related to lower self-esteem, not due to a chronic illness but due to the obvious physical side effects, and that these side effects could be related to problems with intimacy and interpersonal relationships.

There is little research available examining the impact of the side effects of prednisone on self-esteem and social intimacy. The literature is lacking in this information therefore the current study is necessary to examine the impact of prednisone use on self-esteem and social intimacy. This study may provide information that is important for physicians as well as patients who are taking prednisone. The current study examined the relationship between prednisone use and self-esteem, social intimacy, and illness intrusion.

Statement of Purpose

The purpose of the current study examined the correlation between prednisone use and self-esteem, social intimacy, and illness intrusion. Research has shown that chronic illness can have an impact on self-esteem and social relationships (Ireys et al., 1994; Meijer et al., 2000). The study sample included a range of diagnosed chronic conditions that are treated with prednisone. The study examined the relationship between prednisone use, self-esteem, social intimacy and illness intrusion.

Importance of the study

Chronic illness can have a significant influence on one's life and relationships. Even more so, taking medication can result in a greater impact on one's self-esteem and social support, beyond that of having an illness alone. All medications have the risk of potential side effects. Prednisone is shown to result in a variety of physical side effects that could interfere with the way one perceives oneself. The current study offers insight into the way prednisone use may relate to self-esteem and social intimacy.

This study provided important information for physicians who are treating their patients with prednisone. Prednisone can result in mood swings and at times the changes in mood are so severe that psychotropic medications may be prescribed (Sklar, 2002). Because of the nature of medications like prednisone, a therapeutic dose results in unpleasant side effects. Many times other coping strategies have to be developed in order to deal with the side effects of prednisone, such as controlling diet, exercise and skin care strategies. Although the side effects of prednisone are unpleasant, they must be tolerated because for many patients, prednisone may be their only option for treatment (Sklar, 2002). Living with unpleasant side effects is a better alternative than coping with a disease that is out of control (Sklar, 2002). The current study provided insight for psychologists and other mental health professionals treating chronically ill individuals being treated with prednisone. This study also normalized the emotional side effects experienced for patient taking prednisone. Finally the current study expanded the literature and provided information that is currently lacking regarding prednisone use in relation to self-esteem, social intimacy, and social intimacy.

CHAPTER 2

LITERATURE REVIEW

Self-Esteem and Coping with Chronic Illness

People suffering with chronic bronchitis (which can lead to chronic obstructive pulmonary disease or COPD) evidence difficulties breathing which can limit mobility. The limitations to physical activity can result in loneliness and depression. Medication becomes an everyday part of life to manage symptoms. COPD can affect a patient's quality of life. Nicolson and Anderson (2003) investigated the quality of life, adjustment to disease, and self-esteem of people suffering from chronic bronchitis. Quality of life was operationalized by looking at social functioning, physical limitations, pain, physical functioning, perception of health, and impact of symptoms (Nicolson & Anderson, 2003).

Participants in this study were diagnosed with chronic bronchitis, were not suffering from any other chronic conditions, and were hospitalized for long periods of time (Nicolson & Anderson, 2003). The information for the study was obtained from focus groups containing five to six participants in each group. Recruitment occurred in two cities and participants for the four focus groups were obtained from referrals from general practitioners. Twenty adults (10 men and 10 women) agreed to participate in the focus groups. Each group lasted 90 minutes and was tape recorded. Participants were given an outline of the topics to be discussed.

Findings demonstrated that physical symptoms (such as difficulty breathing) contribute to physical as well as psychological distress. Participants reported loss of confidence and social isolation from being chronically ill. Being unable to maintain a social life had a negative impact on quality of life and self-esteem. Participants also reported that embarrassment from the constant coughing negatively impacted self-esteem (Nicolson & Anderson, 2003). Participants reported that both a loss of sense of self and self-blame negatively impacted self-esteem. A sense of loss was experienced by participants because they felt they could not live a normal life. Participants also reported a sense of being a burden to others because they could not fulfill their expected roles. The authors concluded that chronic illness has implications for both physical and psychological well being. This study provided data to support that chronic illness can negatively impact self-esteem.

Multiple Sclerosis (MS) is a chronic illness which has symptoms including weakness, loss of muscle control, slurred speech and incontinence. The symptoms are embarrassing and therefore may have an impact on self-esteem. Walsh and Walsh (1987) evaluated 113 patients with MS in Southern Idaho. Self-esteem was measured using the Rosenberg Self-Esteem Scale. Data were also collected in response to statements about their disease and questions about physical restriction. Those with the lowest level of self-esteem had the most physical restrictions (Walsh & Walsh, 1987). Those with the highest self-esteem had the least physical restrictions (Walsh & Walsh, 1987). This study concluded there was a relationship between self-esteem and level of physical restrictions.

Evidence suggests that patients suffering from chronic illness experienced more emotional well being when they reported higher levels of self-esteem, self-efficacy and social support. Hesselink, Penninx, Schlosser, Wijnhoven, van der Windt, Kriegsman, and van Eijk (2004) examined individual reports on the health related quality of life (HRQoL), coping styles, and coping resources (self-efficacy, self-esteem, mastery and social support) in people with COPD and asthma. Patients with COPD experience difficulty breathing, which reduces their ability level over time. Patients with asthma experience restricted airflow but have periods of remission.

Participants were recruited from 14 doctors in the Netherlands. Participants were diagnosed with either COPD or asthma. The study was completed by 273 patients (220 patients with asthma and 53 patients with COPD). Patients with COPD were older and had less education compared to the patients with asthma. Patients with COPD had also been suffering from the illness longer than patients with asthma. Participants received a questionnaire via mail.

Self-efficacy has been defined as a person's ability to cope with a stressful or unexpected situation, and was measured by the 34 item Self-Efficacy Scale. Mastery defined as the amount of perceived control a person has over his or her life, was measured by the five item Pearlin Mastery Scale. Self-esteem was measured by a response to the statement 'On the whole, I'm satisfied with myself' (Hesselink et al. 2004, p.511) in eight possible life circumstances. Social support was measured by the 12 item Social Support List- Interactions. Three different copings styles were defined. The avoidant or passive coping style was defined as avoiding or denying the seriousness of a problem. The rational or problem focused coping style was defined as changing the situation that is causing problems. The emotional coping style was defined as a passive emotional response. HRQoL reflected the influence the illness has over performance using the Quality of Life in Respiratory Illness Questionnaire (Hesselink et al. 2004).

Patients with COPD reported lower levels of self-efficacy, mastery and self-esteem and had a higher score of emotional coping styles and a lower rating on the HRQoL than patients with asthma (Hesselink et al. 2004). The higher scores of the patients with asthma may be due to the fact that they have more control over their illness if they avoid exertion and take medications properly, which is not the case for COPD. In the case of both patients with COPD or asthma, higher score of emotional coping styles were associated with lower HRQoL scores. Patients with asthma who reported less self-efficacy and less mastery reported lower levels of HRQoL. The authors proposed that avoidant coping styles lead to lower HRQoL. Evidence from this study supports that lowered self-esteem can result from the various side effects of chronic illness. Patients with more limitations in their daily lives had lower self-esteem. Chronic illness can affect a person at any stage of life, from childhood to adolescence to adulthood.

Adolescence is a time of personal and psychological development. Jacobson, Hauser, Powers and Noam (1984) examined self-esteem and ego development in adolescents with diabetes, psychiatric illness, and a control group. Ego development was assessed using the Loevinger Washington University Sentence Completion Test. Self-esteem was evaluated using the Coopersmith Self-Esteem Inventory. The authors were interested in assessing how self-esteem can help aid one's ability to cope.

Jacobson et al. (1984) found no differences in self-esteem between the diabetic group and the control group. Yet, studies with adults with chronic illnesses have shown that self-esteem is lower in adults with increased symptomotology (Walsh & Walsh, 2001). Perhaps age may be a factor influencing the relationship between chronic illness and self-esteem. The limitations of only using adolescents could have contributed to results that differ from what the current study predicts. Adolescents are still developing their self-esteem and the results of the current study were expected to differ from these previous results as the current study evaluated adults.

Chronic illness can have an impact on one's autonomy and independence which can have an impact on self-esteem. Illness symptoms and treatment can interfere with daily activities. Covino, Dirks, Kinsman, and Seidel (1982) examined 132 participants that were depressed and had asthma, tuberculosis, or pain. The participants were required to have a score of greater than 70 on the MMPI depression subscale to be included in the study. Participants ranged from ages 26 to 57 years. Participants were given the MMPI within the first two weeks of hospital admission.

Covino et al. (1982) found that patients with asthma suffered the lowest self-esteem when compared to patients with tuberculosis or pain. Further their lowered self-esteem contributed to feelings of depression. Covino et al. (1982) did not indicate why there was a difference in self-esteem between patients with asthma, tuberculosis, or pain. Patients' depression presented in many different forms. Men reported fewer problems with self-esteem and anxiety than women across all three groups. But the underreporting may be due to cultural and gender pressures than actual self-esteem. Patients with asthma may have reported lower self-esteem due to the treatment of asthma. Prednisone is a common treatment for asthma and perhaps these lower levels of self-esteem could be attributed to prednisone treatment. The current study looked at the relationship between prednisone and self-esteem of participants with a chronic illness.

High self-esteem could be a protective factor against stress and conversely low self-esteem can be associated with depression. Ireys, Gross, Wethamer-Larsson, and Kolodner (1994) looked at self-esteem and impact of illness on social relationships in young adults with a chronic illness. Two hundred and eighty-six participants from Children with Special Health Care Needs in Illinois and Ohio, ranging from ages 20 to

24, participated in the study. Participants had a medical condition for more than a year which required regular medical attention. The three most common disorders were congenital, musculoskeletal and nervous system or sensory disorders. Participants' self-esteem was evaluated using the Rosenberg Self-Esteem Scale. Functional limitations were assessed using Restrictions in Daily Life Index. Two items assessed characteristics of illness course. Participants were also asked to identify other conditions, visibility of condition, vision or hearing problems. Participants were also asked about the perceived impact of an illness on social relationships.

The mean score for all participants on the Rosenberg Self-Esteem Scale was 30.84, indicating moderately high self-esteem. Yet 26% of the sample had scores of less than 28, which the researchers determined indicted low self-esteem. The means for high and low were determined by examining prior studies of adolescents with a chronic illness which had an overall mean of 30.80 and the means for healthy adolescents were between 30.20 and 34.40 (Kellerman, Zeltzer, Ellenberg, Dash & Rigler, 1980). Participants with more than two weeks of restricted activity had lower self-esteem. Participants who had to monitor for sudden changes in condition or who had a deteriorating condition reported lower self-esteem (Ireys et al., 1994). Participants who reported high levels of perceived impact on social relationships reported lower levels of self-esteem. Only 26% of the participants in the study by Ireys et al. (1994) reported an impact of low self-esteem that affected various aspects of life, including social relationships. Although the results of this study only resulted in one quarter of the participants reporting lower self-esteem, the impact of low self-esteem in people with chronic illness affected various areas of life.

Long term effect of chronic illness and self-esteem

Children and adolescents with chronic illness report low body image, low self-esteem and problems with behavior. There is a higher risk of psychological problems with diseases with an uncertain course, chronic pain and conditions that are not visible. Huurre and Aro (2002) conducted a longitudinal study examining the psychological well being of chronically ill individuals at ages 16, 22, and 32.

The participants were contacted in southern Finland in 1983, 1989 and 1999 and asked to fill out a questionnaire. Fifty-two participants reported a chronic illness that affected their everyday life, 244 participants reported a chronic illness that did not limit their daily life, and 401 participants reported no chronic illness. There were more women than men in the chronic illness group. The chronic illnesses represented in this study were asthma, allergies, skin allergies, allergic rhinitis, migraines and diabetes. Participants were administered a variety of questionnaires and a checklist of somatic complaints. A self-esteem scale modified for Finnish students was used. The General Health Questionnaire was used to evaluate psychological distress. Participants completed the short 13 item Beck Depression Inventory and the Alcohol Use Disorders Identification Test. Social support was evaluated by Vaux and Harrison's (1985) Social Support Resources.

Adults with limiting chronic illness were less likely to be married or living with someone, when compared to healthy individuals and participants whose chronic illness were not limiting. Adults with chronic illness were not different from healthy participants in education, employment or SES. Participants with limiting chronic illness were more depressed and had lower self-esteem than healthy individuals. Chronic illness did not prevent people from engaging in unhealthy behaviors, like smoking. This study also indicates that chronic illness may negatively impact social and intimate relationships. The current study evaluated if medication use has an impact on self-esteem and social relationships.

Following a myocardial infarction (MI), self-care behaviors such as exercise, smoking cessation, adhering to medications, dietary modification and stress management are essential to preventing future problems. Self-esteem and social support seem to help patients succeed at healthy self-care behaviors. A decrease in self-esteem inhibits people from adhering to the medical guidelines. Conn, Taylor, and Hayes (1992) examined the relationship between self-care behaviors and self-esteem and social support following a MI.

A nonrandom sample of 117 men and 80 women who were over the age of 40 and survived an MI were given a questionnaire. Multiple chronic illnesses were common and 89 of the participants were active smokers. Social support was measured by the Personal Resources Questionnaire (PRQ) and self-esteem was measured by the Rosenberg Self-Esteem Scale. The 20 item Health Behavior Scale assessed how well the patient adhered to his or her medical prescriptions.

Self-esteem was related to self-care behaviors such as exercise, diet and stress management. Adhering to medication was predicted by social support but not self-esteem. Self-esteem and social support significantly predicted exercise. Although smoking was not affected by self-esteem or social support, elimination of smoking was the single most important predictor of post MI mortality (Conn, Taylor, & Hayes, 1992). This study is an example of self-esteem as a predictor of self-care behaviors such as exercise, diet and stress management. It is important to maintain a healthy self-esteem in order to assure adherence to medical recommendations such as self-care behaviors and taking medication properly. Maintaining one's health and having healthy self-esteem could lead to positive interpersonal relationships.

Self-Image and Chronic Illness

Chronic illness can affect every aspect of someone's life, from self-esteem (satisfaction with one's self) to self-image (concept of one's self). Erkolahti, Ilonen, and Saarijarvi (2003) compared the self-image of adolescents with diabetes mellitus and rheumatoid arthritis. In the study, 74 adolescents were studied, 23 with diabetes, 25 with arthritis, and 26 controls, who were matched for age, sex, and SES. Participants were identified from hospital records from Turku University Central Hospital in Turku, Finland. The participants with diabetes had their illness under good control and the participants with arthritis were functioning at a medium level.

The Offer Self-Image Questionnaire (OSIQ) was used to assess impulse control, emotional tone, body image, social relations, vocational and educational goals, sexual attitudes, family relations, mastery of the external world, emotional health and superior adjustment (Erkolahti et al. 2003).

Erkolahti et al. (2003) found that the adolescents with diabetes or arthritis had higher scores than the control group on impulse control, emotional tone, social relations, sexual attitudes, family relations, mastery of external world, emotional health and superior adjustment. These higher scores showed that the arthritis group had better control of their lives and relationships. Adolescents who were chronically ill had lower scores on body image and vocational and educational goals than the controls (Erkolahti et al. 2003). The study found no significant differences between the self-image of adolescents with arthritis and diabetes when compared with the controls. Patients with arthritis reported good self-esteem when their impairment was moderate (Erkolahti et al. 2003). The lowered scores on body image could be attributed to their concern for their health and not being proud of their bodies (Erkolahti et al. 2003). This study did not specify what medications, if any, were taken by the adolescents. The current study specifically focused on prednisone use.

Although the patients with arthritis reported good self-esteem, it is also important to note that their impairment was moderate. If they were more affected by their illness, their self-esteem scores may have been different. This study also found that participants with a chronic illness had lower body image than the controls. The physical side effects of prednisone may alter one's appearance, which could distort the way a person perceives himself or herself and could therefore contribute to a diminished body image. Prednisone use may have a relationship with self-esteem and social intimacy and the current study evaluated that relationship.

Self-esteem and autonomy

Litt, Cuskey, and Rosenberg (1982) looked at the relationship between self-esteem and autonomy on the medication compliance of adolescents with Juvenile Rheumatoid Arthritis. Noncompliance to salicylate treatment is associated with earlier onset of the disease and longer disease duration. Self-concept was important to the study because noncompliance is high for adolescents who are prescribed steroids which have a negative effect on appearance.

Thirty-eight adolescents from the Arthritis Clinic at Children's Hospital at Stanford during 1978 and 1979 were part of a longitudinal study. The mean age of the group was 14.2. Thirty-nine percent of the participants were male and 61% were female and all the participants were Caucasian (Litt et al., 1982). The participants completed the 80 item Piers-Harris Self-concept scale and the five item Autonomy scale developed by Eysenk (1975). Compliance was measured by serum salicylate levels over 12 months.

Compliant patients scored significantly higher on the self-concept scale than those who were not compliant (Litt et al., 1982). Compliant patients perceived themselves as autonomous and took more responsibility for their healthcare. The hypothesis that a positive self-image and compliance are associated was supported. Higher self-esteem was reported in patients who were less ill at the onset of their illness.

Self-image is an important component in patients' compliance to recommended medical regimens (Litt et al., 1982). Self-image or the way one views oneself can have an impact on self-esteem. If patient's self-esteem is lowered due to medication side effects, the patient may be less likely to adhere to medical prescriptions. Prednisone has many physical side effects that can contribute to lowering one's self-esteem. If patients suffer from lower self-esteem, they may not take their prescriptions as directed, which may result in further physical complications.

<u>Chronic Illness and Social Support</u>

The diagnosis of cancer can be devastating especially for patients with ovarian cancer. Ovarian cancer is often caught in an advanced stage therefore patients have a poor prognosis. Surgery can cause harm to body image and recurrence rates of cancer are 30 to 50 percent (Rubin et al., 1991). Much of the psychological stress that is encountered is due to physical impairment from either the disease or treatment. One of the most influential sources of stress is from unsupportive or aversive reactions from family and friends. Unsupportive responses are characterized as being critical, avoiding the topic of cancer, and minimizing the effects of cancer (Norton, Manne, Hernandez, Rubin, & Carlson, 2005). People suffering from a life threatening illness look to friends and family for validation and lack of validation can impact their self-esteem (Norton et al., 2005).

Norton et al. (2005) evaluated 143 women diagnosed with ovarian cancer. The average age was 55 and most participants were married for an average of 27.8 years. The mean length since diagnosis was 18 months. Seventy-six percent of participants were currently receiving chemotherapy.

Participants completed the Functional Status of the Cancer Rehabilitation Evaluation System to assess physical impairment. Participants completed the 13-item Perceived Negative Behaviors Scale to evaluate unsupportive or negative behaviors of friends and family. Items adapted from Thompson et al. (1993) were used to evaluate participants' perceived control over their illness. The Rosenberg Self Esteem Scale was used to assess self-esteem. The 12-item Psychological Distress Scale of the Mental Health Inventory- 18(MHI-18) was used to examine anxiety, depression and loss of behavioral and emotional control not due to illness specifically.

The study found that higher levels of physical impairment were associated with lower levels of control over one's illness. Higher levels of unsupportive behaviors from family and friends were associated with lower levels of self-esteem which contributed to more psychological distress. The negative view of family and friends can result in feeling of rejection which in turn leads to lower self-esteem (Norton et al., 2005). People with chronic illnesses are hypersensitive to the possibility of social isolation which may make them vulnerable to allowing unsupportive behaviors to affect self-esteem (Druely & Townsend, 1998). Interventions with cancer patients should focus on improving one's feelings of control over an illness and to improve self-esteem in response to negative family behaviors (Norton et al., 2005).

The study by Norton et al. (2005) shows the importance of the support of family and friends during times of illness. Socially intimate relationships are important during times of stress. The support of family and friends can bolster or hinder self-esteem and is therefore important during times of illness.

For some people, the threat of a chronic illness is enough to induce significant stress. A quarter of a million women a year in England and Wales seek medical advice for a lump in their breast, and only 30,000 of those cases result in a diagnosis of breast cancer (McPherson, Steel & Dixon, 2000). Many women experience unnecessary stress prior to their appointments. Social support is also an important factor in reducing stress. Spousal support helps reduce all life stressors and friend support was shown to reduce the stress of health problems (Jackson, 1992). Married women are less likely to get sick and have lower mortality rates than their single counterparts (Gale et al., 2001). Yet the quality of the relationship is important as well.

Gale et al. (2001) evaluated 158 women who were referred to a breast clinic at a hospital to have a lump examined. Of the 158 women, 118 had a partner and of those 118 with a partner, 40 of them did not live with their partner. Participants completed the Global Measure of Perceived Stress, the Hospital Anxiety and Depression Scale, and

Culture Free SEI Self-Esteem Inventories for Children and Adults. Social support was measured by the Significant Other Scale. The quality of the relationship with one's partner was evaluated by the Dyadic Adjustment Scale. The surveys were administered twice, once one to four days before the diagnostic appointment and again while waiting to see the doctor.

Some patients reported high levels of stress (26.5%), anxiety (28.5%), and depression (3.2%) immediately before their appointment (Gale et al., 2001). The levels of stress and depression were lower on the day of the appointment, which was unexpected. Women with a partner had a lower stress level on the day of the appointment than women without a partner. Women with a lower quality relationship experienced more stress than those with a supportive partner (Gale et al., 2001). Women's level of self-esteem was not related to having a partner or the quality of the relationship. Yet, self-esteem was the best predictor of stress. A majority of the women in this study were given a benign diagnosis. One-third of the women who received a diagnosis of cancer experienced long term distress which could affect their adjustment to an illness as well as their health (Gale et al., 2001).

Managing a chronic illness in a family setting can be challenging. Many illnesses are managed through dietary restrictions, which can be problematic for the family. Many family social engagements involve food therefore dietary restrictions can cause some difficulty. Gregory (2005) looked at the impact of families coping with chronic illness that involve dietary guidelines. Gregory (2005) interviewed families affected by coronary heart disease (CHD) and celiac disease (CD). Coronary heart disease is a well-known illness with dietary guidelines as one form of treatment. CHD diet recommendations involve eating healthy by lowering cholesterol and by losing weight. Celiac disease is a little known condition that is solely treated with dietary restrictions such as excluding gluten from the diet. Gluten is used in nearly all food products including flour, bread, and pasta and is quite challenging to eliminate.

For many individuals, chronic illness is a medical condition that is restricted more by social consequences than by the impact of physical symptoms or treatment (Gregory, 2005). Food and dining rituals are many times a large part of normal familial interactions. The restrictions on diet can disrupt these social and nutritional interactions. Gregory (2005) looked at the impact of diet restricted illness on families specifically the main care taker responsible for food preparation.

The study was conducted in southern England with 13 males with CHD, six females with CHD, 10 males with CD and 12 females with CD (Gregory, 2005). The study was conducted by doing a series of interviews with the family members. A total of 61 people were interviewed from 41 families. All of the relationships were heterosexual and only five families did not have children. Most of the children in the families studied no longer lived at home. Of the CD group 14 were employed and eight were unemployed. Of the CHD group three were employed and 16 were unemployed. The purpose of this study was not to determine how effectively patients have maintained their diets, but to see the impact of diet on the family.

The diagnosis of an illness is not a turning point but the start of an ongoing process of adjustment and care (Gregory, 2005). Participants with CD were more likely to have experienced symptoms over a lifetime, where participants with CHD were more likely to have sudden symptoms. Many participants told their doctors that they believed they would be able to lead a normal life and the patients with CD reported about a one year adjustment to dietary restrictions followed by a return to somewhat normal life.

The study showed that families had to make ongoing adjustments to chronic illness and dietary restrictions. There was a familial need to restore normalcy as much as possible following a diagnosis. The onset of illness can change gender roles and the roles in the family. Maintaining gender identity and family identity was important to the person with the chronic illness. Most participants could adhere to dietary recommendations while maintaining gender roles. The study by Gregory (2005) shows how families are affected by chronic illness yet strive to maintain normalcy, although it is unclear if that was achieved. Chronic illness impacts every aspect of life and the current study will extend the literature to examine how a treatment of chronic illness, specifically prednisone, relates to two aspects of life, self-esteem and social intimacy.

Adjustment to chronic illness can be made increasingly difficult when family and medical staff do not understand the magnitude of an illness. Hatchett, Friend, Symister and Wadhwa (1997) looked at the patient and familial expectations surrounding end stage renal dialysis care. There were three areas of familial and medical staff expectations that were examined including: coping with the illness, responsibility for one's treatment, and ability to execute everyday functions (Hatchett et al., 1997). Hatchett et al.(1997) concluded that the inability to meet the expectations of others, in regard to one's illness, may result in depression. Many of the patients studied with renal disease suffered from anemia which left the patient weak and fatigued. Findings suggest, many families have difficulty understanding the limitations of invisible symptoms, such as fatigue.

Patients with end stage renal disease were recruited from a large university hospital. Sixty-eight patients completed the first questionnaires at Time 1 and three months later at Time 2, 42 patients completed the second set of questionnaires. At Time 2, 11 patients had died, six had transferred hospitals and nine declined completing the second questionnaire. The patients' mean age was 56, and 50% were men. The mean time on dialysis was 4.4 years. Patients completed an 11 item questionnaire developed by the researchers to assess perceptions of family and friends expectations (Hatchett et al., 1997). Hatchett et al. (1997) also developed a seven item measure to examine the patients' perception of medical staff expectations. Ten items of the Inventory of Socially Supportive Behaviors (Barrera, Sandler, & Ramsey, 1981) assessed perceived medical social support. Ten items adapted from the Dialysis Regimen Scale of Social Support (Whitaker, 1989) assessed perceived family and friends' social support. Social desirability was assessed using Reynolds (1982) short form of the Marlowe-Crowne Social Desirability Scale. Participants also completed the Beck Depression Inventory, the Hopelessness Scale evaluating hopelessness about the future, and the Illness Effects Questionnaire.

Patients who experienced difficulties with familial expectations perceived lower social support. Three constructs were moderately correlated: depression, hopelessness and quality of life (Hatchett et al., 1997). The Family Expectation Scale resulted in a significant correlation with depression and somewhat weaker, yet statistically significant correlations with hopelessness, illness intrusion, and quality of life (Hatchett et al., 1997). Patients who felt they were unable to meet the expectations of their family and medical staff were more likely to experience depression, intrusion from illness, and poorer quality of life, regardless of the perceived social support (Hatchett, et al., 1997).

Family and medical staff may lack knowledge or comprehension about chronic illness and its effects, which may cause patients to perceive the expectations of others as unreasonable. Patients' perceptions of family expectations had more impact on patients' depression than perceived medical staff expectations. However, perceived medical staff expectations were related to hopelessness. The patients' self-esteem may be affected by perceived or actual physical limitations. People may feel inadequate when they are not able to participate or perform as expected. Understanding interpersonal expectations can help patients adjust and may improve psychological well-being.

Chronic illnesses can have an impact on marital interactions. Chronic illnesses result in changes in finances and household responsibilities and these stressors can have a negative impact on marital relationships (Badr & Actitelli, 2005). Carter and Carter (1994) recruited patients with Parkinson's disease (PD) and their spouses. Forty-six couples participated, 35 males and 11 females with PD. The mean age of the spouses was 65.7 years and the mean for length of marriage was 39.3 years. Participants were separated into two groups, 20 patients with PD and chronically ill spouses and 26 patients with PD and well spouses. Chronically ill spouses suffered from cardiovascular disease, arthritis, asthma, cancer, and diabetes. The Dyadic Adjustment Scale was used to measure martial adjustment and Projective Sentence Completion was used to evaluate the effects of illness.

Carter and Carter (1994) found that marital adjustments and disability were not significantly related, suggesting that spouses' appraisal of marital adjustment was unrelated to disability. The difference between spouses' and patients' martial adjustment scores was not statistically significant, which suggests that level of marital adjustment is similar regardless of illness. Patients with PD and their chronically ill spouses identify that the illness had a positive effect on the marriage. More well spouses than patients reported negative effects of PD on the marriage. Patients with chronically ill spouses reported worrying about the illness, had better relationships with physicians, and positive interactions with spouse and communicating about the future. Patients with well spouses reported a negative relationship with physicians and friends. Over half of the well spouses reported negative marital interactions due to illness where only five ill spouses reported negative interactions due to disease (Carter & Carter, 1994). Half of the ill spouses reported changes in life as a result of illness but half of the well spouses reported no life changes.

Although not specifically assessed in the study by Carter and Carter (1994), understanding of illness effects can have a major impact on the way one copes with chronic illness in one's spouse. Chronically ill spouses could relate to and understand the chronic illness of their partners which may have established a bond and lessened the perception of the negative effects of PD on their relationship.

Rheumatoid arthritis (RA) is an autoimmune disease resulting in pain, fatigue and disfiguration. Patients with RA have difficulty coping with the unpredictable nature of the illness. Many patients' families have difficulty understanding RA which can make adjustment to the disease difficult. Bediako and Friend (2004) looked at perceived expectations of family and friends of patients with RA.

Thirty-nine women and their spouses participated in the study. The mean age of the women was 46.9 years with mean disease duration of 11 years. Participants completed a Perceived Expectation Scale to evaluate the perceived expectations from significant others. Social support and problematic relations were assessed using the Positive and Problematic Support Scale. Relationship quality was evaluated using the Dyadic Adjustment Scale. Perceived criticism of family and friends and disease severity were assessed. Depression was evaluated using the Beck Depression Inventory. Patients' perceived expectations and spouses' demands were highly correlated. Patients who felt unable to meet the demands of their spouse also had fewer social support behaviors, lower relationship quality and more problematic interactions (Bediako & Friend, 2004). Patients who felt unable to meet the expectations of their spouse also felt misunderstood by their spouse. Positive social support, problematic relations, and perceived criticism were not related to depression. This study shows how the impact of chronic illness can affect intimate relationships.

Intimate Relationships and Social Support

Physical illness can have a negative impact on a person's self-worth and self-esteem. Marital interactions have direct impact on one's sense of well being. Druley and Townsend (1998) proposed that positive marital interaction would be associated with less depression and higher self-esteem and negative marital interactions would be associated with more depression and lower self-esteem. The data were analyzed from the Americans' Changing Lives (ACL) survey in 1986 in which 3,617 people participated in interviews averaging 86 minutes. The group used in the study was under 50 because the authors proposed that illness causes more distress for younger couples (Coyne & Smith,

1991). Two groups were selected, 90 individuals with arthritis and 90 individuals without arthritis or any other illnesses were selected to match the arthritis group on age, income, gender and length of marriage. There were 37 men and 53 women in each group. The group with arthritis reported limitations to daily activities and being less satisfied with their health. Positive and negative marital interactions were assessed by answering six items. Self-esteem was assessed by giving four items from the Rosenberg Self-Esteem Scale. In order to assess depression, eight items were taken from the Center for Epidemiologic Studies Depression Scale.

Positive and negative marital interactions were separate scales and analyzed independently. For both groups, positive marital interactions and higher self-esteem were related to fewer symptoms of depression (Druely & Townsend, 1998). Yet for both groups, positive marital interactions were not related to self-esteem. The group of participants with arthritis did not report an increase in negative marital interaction when compared to the control group. Yet negative marital interactions were related to lower self-esteem for the participants with arthritis. However, negative marital interactions were not related to depression for either group. The study by Druely and Townsend (1998), found a relationship between negative marital interactions and self-esteem.

Social support is an important component when coping with a chronic illness. Symister and Friend (2003) hypothesized that support would be associated with depression and optimism, and that self-esteem would mediate that interaction. Symister and Friend (2003) believed that social support would lead to better self-esteem which would be related to lower depression and higher optimism. Symister and Friend (2003) also believed that negative interactions would lead to lower self-esteem, higher depression and lower optimism.

Participants were patients with end-stage renal disease (ESRD) recruited from five hospitals or dialysis centers in New York City. Data were collected initially and again three months later. One hundred and fifty eight participants completed the first set of surveys and 86 participants returned three months later for the second series of questionnaires. Social support was measured by the 40 item Interpersonal Support Evaluation List (ISEL) which measures appraisal support, tangible support, self-esteem support, and belonging support (Symister & Friend, 2003). Problematic support was measured by the 40 item Inventory of Negative Social Interactions. Optimism was measured using the 10 item Life Orientation Test-Revised. Participants also completed the Rosenberg Self-Esteem Scale, Beck Depression Inventory and the Positive- Negative Affect Schedule.

Self-esteem mediated the relationship between depression and optimism and social support. Social support was important for reducing depression as well as increasing self-esteem. Problematic support was not related to self-esteem. Belonging support assessed how accessible other people are for social interaction and the degree the participant was able to interact socially which was important in increasing optimism and decreasing depression. Tangible support from others was also related to increased self-esteem and optimism. The results were surprising, finding that problematic support had no effect on self-esteem.

Emotional support and positive self-esteem can help when coping with a chronic illness. Authors have examined whether cultural influences affect support and coping with a chronic illness. Cultural attitudes and belief systems may influence one's optimal level of support and effective coping. For instance, maintaining family roles is an important part of Latino culture. Abraido-Lanza (2004) investigated how too much social support when coping with arthritis can jeopardize a Latina's feeling of usefulness as a homemaker.

Ninety-eight Latina women were selected to participate. All of the women had rheumatic disease and had listed homemaker as central to their identity. The women participated in a structured interview developed by the Stanford Patient Education Research Center for the Spanish Arthritis Self Management Program (SASMP) (Avraido-Lanza, 2004). Pain was measured by the Medical Outcome Study measurement and disability was measured by the Health Assessment Questionnaire (HAQ). Identifying the importance of the homemaker role was surveyed by a subscale of Luhtanen and Crocker's Collective Self-esteem Scale. Emotional support was evaluated by a measure designed specifically for arthritis patients. Participants completed Rosenberg Self-Esteem Scale and the Positive and Negative Affect Schedule (PANAS). Self-efficacy was also assessed.

About one-third of the women reported positive feelings toward receiving help with the housework, but only if that help was from a female member of the family. Yet another one third reported negative feeling about receiving help with the housework. Support was beneficial to self-esteem if the support was from an appropriate source, a female family member. Many respondents reported unpleasant feelings if their spouse helped with the housework. The study showed that support led to less psychological distress if the support was from an appropriate female family member, which may be culturally bound. Chronic illness can affect one's self-esteem as well as one's self-concept. Social support is an important factor to maintaining a positive outlook. Being able to have intimate contact with a spouse or a family member to receive social support could contribute to positive self-esteem.

Multiple sclerosis (MS) is a chronic neurological disease that can impact self-esteem and psychological adjustment. Due to the incapacitation caused by MS, the disease has an impact on one's quality of life. Studies have shown a strong relationship between social support and self-esteem with people with MS (Foote et al., 1990). The study by McCabe and Di Battista (2004), investigated the relationships between health variables, social relationships, work, coping, psychological adjustment and self-esteem of people with MS and compared them to the general population.

The random sample of people with MS consisted of 251 participants from the MS Society of Victoria, Australia, ranging from 18-65 years old. The general population consisted of a random sample of 184 participants drawn from the electoral poll, ranging in age from 21-65 years old. Participants completed the World Health Organization Quality of Life- 100 scale to assess work ability, health and social relationships. Participants were also given the Profile of Mood States-Short Form that is a list of adjectives to assess for tension, depression, and confusion. Participants also completed the 30-item Folkman and Lazarus's Ways of Coping Questionnaire to assess for coping strategies. Participants completed the set of questionnaires twice, 18 months apart.

Participants with MS reported higher levels of anxiety, depression, confusion and lower levels of self-esteem (McCabe & Di Battista, 2004). Compared to the general population, participants with MS had lower levels of mobility, social relationships, and work ability and higher levels of pain (McCabe & Di Battista, 2004). Participants with MS reported lower levels of coping, seeking social support and higher levels of detachment (McCabe & Di Battista, 2004). There were no significant gender differences for either group of participants. Levels of self-esteem and adjustment were stable for people with MS over the 18 month period. This stability could be due to lack of coping and seeking social support. Perhaps if participants sought social support, their psychological well-being and self-esteem might improve. The current study examined the relationship between prednisone use, self-esteem, social intimacy and illness intrusion.

Illness Intrusiveness

Multiple sclerosis (MS) is an autoimmune disease that results in the destruction of myelin in the central nervous system. MS results in loss of functioning which can be painful as well as stressful. Illness intrusion is the degree in which the illness and treatment disrupts lifestyle. Illness uncertainty is due to the unpredictable nature of the illness and lack of a cure. Mullins, Cote, Fuemmeler, Jean, Beatty, and Paul (2001) looked at illness intrusiveness and illness uncertainty with people with MS.

Seventy-eight participants with MS participated in the study. Nine were taking corticosteroids, like prednisone, at the time of the study. The Ambulation Index measured disability. Illness intrusion was evaluated using the Illness Intrusiveness Scale. Illness intrusiveness measures the way illness and treatment disrupts activities, well-being and quality of life (Devins et al., 2001). The Mishel Uncertainty in Illness-Community Form was used to measure illness uncertainty. Illness uncertainty is the unpredictability of one's illness, treatment and prognosis (Mishel & Braden, 1988). The Symptom Checklist-90 Revised was used to evaluate psychological distress.

Illness intrusiveness and illness uncertainty were significant predictors of psychological adjustment (Mullins et al. 2001). Illness intrusiveness can affect one's psychological adjustment which can impact various areas of life. The current study evaluated if illness intrusion is more significant for participants taking prednisone than for participants with a chronic illness that are not taking prednisone.

The Effects of Steroid Use

Corticosteroids, like prednisone, can result in psychiatric and cognitive side effects (Naude & Pretorious, 2003). Glucocorticoids (e.g. prednisone) are used to treat many inflammation illnesses such as lupus, asthma and inflammatory bowel disease (Keenan & Kuhn, 1999). Glucocorticoids can disrupt cognition which may be due to hippocampal dysfunction. Glucocorticoids can impair memory by decreasing the glucose uptake into the hippocampus. The hippocampus is vital for encoding new information. Prednisone has more than just physical side effects; memory side effects are reported as well. There is evidence for declining memory due to prednisone use (Keenan & Kuhn, 1999). Patients treated with prednisone (mean dose of 15mg a day) showed impairment on paragraph recall tests after only one year of treatment (Keenan & Kuhn, 1999). Memory was more affected by length of use rather than dosage. Even short term use of three months had an adverse effect on memory. Prednisone is commonly used to treat childhood asthma, and patients with asthma have shown deficits in visual and verbal memory. The damage to one's memory could perhaps result in lower self-esteem because of lack of confidence in one's ability.

Many side effects can result from steroids. Weight gain is an adverse side effect of steroids which can leave women at a risk of developing an eating disorder. Fornari, Dancyger, La Monaca, Budman, Goodman, Kabo, and Katz (2001) looked at eight case reports of women who were prescribed prednisone and developed an eating disorder. In these eight cases of women prescribed a steroid, two developed anorexia nervosa, five developed bulimia nervosa, and one developed an eating disorder not otherwise specified in response to the weight gain. These women received psychological treatment for their eating disorders.

According to the *Diagnostic and statistical manual of mental disorders, text revision* (American Psychiatric Association, 2000) 0.5% of the population will develop anorexia nervosa and 1-3% or the population will develop bulimia nervosa. Fornari et al. (2001) found that of the people that developed an eating disorder, 2% of people who presented in the eating disorder clinic were prescribed a steroid shortly before the onset of an eating disorder. Statistics were not available regarding the number of people who are prescribed prednisone that also develop an eating disorder. Three of the cases had a history of being overweight and five of the cases had a co-morbid Axis I diagnosis in addition to an eating disorder. Although it is a small percentage of patients with an eating disorder who were treated with steroids, it is still important for physicians and psychologists to be aware of the possible risk factors of developing an eating disorder following steroid use. People with long term problems with self-esteem and weight may be more susceptible to develop an eating disorder as Fornari et al. (2001) has shown. The use of steroids may effect the body's appearance which can have an impact on self-esteem. The current study investigated the relationship between prednisone use, self-esteem, and social intimacy.

Perceived Medication Side Effects

Upon receiving a medical prescription, many patients receive a list of possible side effects. These side effects could impact whether a patient chooses to take the medication prescribed. The study by Berry, Michas, and Bersellini (2002) looked at the perceived risk of side effects and the possible influence on prescription adherence. Three different hypothetical situations were examined.

The first experiment examined the approximated likelihood that compliance was affected by information about side effects. The experiment also surveyed perceived risk and satisfaction. In the first experiment, 976 healthy volunteers (450 males and 526 females) were recruited from local shopping areas and clubs. Each participant was given a booklet describing a hypothetical situation of being diagnosed with an illness and being prescribed a medication. The scenarios differed based on severity of disease (mild or severe), the severity of the side effect (mild or severe), the likelihood the side effects would occur (likely or unlikely) and the number of side effects (few or many) (Berry et al., 2002). Participants were instructed to read the booklets and answer the questions pertaining to the hypothetical situation described.

Perceived satisfaction, risk to health, and probability of experiencing side effects was affected by age; the oldest group gave the highest ratings on these three categories (Berry et al., 2002). The youngest group gave the highest rating on intention to comply. The high anxiety group had a higher rating of risk to health, reported higher levels of disease severity and a higher probability of experiencing side effects, as compared to the low anxiety group. Side effect severity was rated highest by the entire sample compared to the impact of likelihood or number of side effects.

The second experiment looked at the negative side effect of a medication and the benefit of taking the medication. In the second experiment, 592 volunteers (282 males and 310 females) were given a scenario describing a hypothetical situation of being diagnosed with an illness and being prescribed a medication. Each of the scenarios differed based on the severity of the side effect (mild or severe), severity of disease (mild or severe), and benefit statement (no statement, positive benefit, or unknown benefit) (Berry et al., 2002). The positive benefit statement said that the medication was effective and would eliminate the disease in three or four days. The unknown benefit statement said that the medication was new and it was unclear how effective it was.

In the second experiment consistent with experiment one, allocated satisfaction, appraisal of the risk to health, and probability of experiencing side effects were affected by age; the oldest group gave the highest ratings on these three categories (Berry et al., 2002). Once again, the youngest group gave the highest rating on intention to comply. The high anxiety group had higher rating of risk to health, disease severity and the probability of experiencing side effects, compared to the low anxiety group. Participants reported greater risk when told they were suffering from a mild illness opposed to a severe illness. The assigned side effect severity caused more variability related to satisfaction for mild diagnosis than severe diagnosis. Higher levels of satisfaction were reported when the medication was known to eliminate the illness. Higher levels of risk and lower levels of compliance were reported in the situation when the medication was new and not yet established.

The third experiment assessed how control over preventing or alleviating the side effects affected compliance. In the third experiment, 515 volunteers (230 males and 285 females) were given a description of a hypothetical situation of being diagnosed with an illness and being prescribed a medication. Each of the possible scenarios differed based on severity of disease (mild or severe), the severity of the side effect (mild or severe), and control statement (no statement, prevention statement, or alleviation statement) (Berry et al., 2002). The prevention statement said that taking the medication correctly would reduce the potential for side effects. The alleviation statement said that if the hypothetical patient experienced side effects and alerted the doctor, that he or she could adjust the dose or recommend a new medication.

The third experiment found that the oldest group gave the highest ratings on satisfaction (Berry et al., 2002). Perhaps the oldest group was more accustomed to taking medication with side effects and was therefore more likely to perceive satisfaction in the hypothetical situation. The prevention statement resulted in participants believing in a lower likelihood of experiencing side effects. The prevention statement also resulted in lower perceived risk and higher reports of compliance (Berry et al., 2002).

Overall, the participants who received a description of negative side effects were less satisfied, perceived risk to be higher and were less likely to adhere to the medical prescription. The greatest impact was caused by the expected side effect severity. Side effects were perceived as less likely to occur but more severe when paired with the mild disease. Participants were more likely to state medication compliance with a severe illness. New and not established medication was less likely to be taken. Telling participants how to reduce the side effects was helpful. Older people were more satisfied but also perceived a higher risk. Young participants were more likely to comply with the medication prescription.

The study by Berry et al. (2002) produced valuable information, but the participants were a group of healthy volunteers. The study examined people's perceptions of hypothetical situations. The study might have been more useful if a population with a diagnosed illness was used. If the participants were currently taking medication, the results may have given a more accurate picture of a patient's reactions to medicinal side effects. This study shows that consideration of side effects affect the perceptions of people regarding their health and their willingness to comply with a medication in a hypothetical situation.

When the side effects were described as severe, participants in the Berry et al. (2002) study were less likely to be satisfied and less likely to adhere to the medications. Due to the side effects of prednisone, people may be less likely to adhere and less satisfied with their treatment. Not adhering to medications can cause further medical complications or force the patient to take prednisone longer, prolonging the negative side effect and reduction in self-esteem. Understanding the expected side effects may help patients prepare for the possible physical changes they may experience.

Most medications can result in some sort of side effect. Side effects can result in patients not wanting to take their medication as prescribed. The physical side effects can be distressing and result in emotional disturbances or disruptions in well being. Bothersome physical side effects can result from prednisone, as well as many other prescriptions, including psychological medications. The literature on psychological medication can provide a foundation for the current hypotheses.

Side Effects of Psychological Medications

Much of the literature available about the consequences of side effects of medication is based in literature on psychological medication. Antipsychotic medication is prescribed to treat schizophrenia, yet many of these medicines produce undesirable side effects, ranging from dry mouth, constipation or stiffness. New atypical antipsychotic drugs have fewer side effects. Carrick, Mitchell, Powell and Lloyd (2004) examined the quest for well-being while taking an antipsychotic medication.

Twenty-five participants (12 women and 13 men) who were taking antipsychotic medication, had a diagnosis of schizophrenia and were between ages 18-65, were included in the study. The study was conducted in two phases; phase I was a focus group and phase II was an individual interview. Participants reported that the side effects and symptoms of illness were road blocks to well-being. Well-being was defined as being able to function normally, feel normal, to function in the world, and to appear normal to everyone else (Carrick et al. 2004). Both the illness and treatment resulted in distress. Patients were prepared to deal with side effects in order to improve.

Women were most concerned with side effects of fatigue and weight gain. Mental side effects also resulted in distress. Some participants complained that their doctors did not provide them with adequate information about the possibility of side effects. Many participants developed coping strategies such as drinking more water to reduce dry mouth. Some people had positive coping strategies such as exercising to minimize weight gain, while others became socially withdrawn. Some side effects were more personally disturbing than others. Participants complained that doctors were not aware of the impact side effects had on well-being. Participants were aware that there might not be a perfect treatment but side effects did present a barrier to achieving well-being (Carrick et al. 2004). The impact of side effects could affect a patients' perception of well-being as was demonstrated by Carrick et al. (2004). Affecting the perceptions of one's well-being could have an impact on their self-esteem. The impact of side effects is distressing to many patients and the current study examined if the side effects of prednisone have a relationship with self-esteem and social intimacy.

Affect and Medication

Asthma is a chronic illness that may require constant medication. Many people use inhaled corticosteroids and short acting beta-agonists together to maintain self-management. Overuse of a beta-agonist can lead to unpleasant side effects such as increased pulse, muscle tremors, and central nervous system stimulation as well as psychological symptoms such as anxiety. Negative affect or negative mood effects patient's interpretation of their asthma, many times causing them to use more medication. Negative affect can result in physical symptoms patients may misinterpret as asthma. Main, Moss-Morris, Booth, Kaptein, and Kolbe (2003) examined whether negative moods influence the way patients label their symptoms as asthma and if they consequently take more medication.

Forty-two participants were recruited from an outpatient asthma clinic in New Zealand. The age of the participants ranged from 19 to 76 and 69% of the participants were women. Participants ranged in duration from having asthma for 3 to 63 years with a mean of 29 years.

Participants filled out a set of questionnaires daily for seven days. Participants completed the Revised Illness Perception Questionnaire which measures beliefs about illness, illness identity and asks if a wide range of symptoms are characteristic of one's illness. The symptom checklist contained items related to asthma, such as tight chest and others unrelated to asthma such as nausea. Participants completed the 20 item Positive Affect and Negative Affect Scales (PANAS). Participants also kept track of how many times they used their reliever in one day. Every evening the participants used a Mini-Wright peak flow meter to record lung function.

At least one-third of the participants labeled symptoms as asthma related even though they were really symptoms of anxiety (Main et al. 2003). Negative affect and incorrect asthma symptom labeling lead to an increase in use of reliever. Less than one-quarter of the participants used their relievers as recommended. Negative affect was correlated with somatic symptoms that were interpreted as asthma. The number of symptoms associated with asthma was related to negative mood. Negative affect lead to an increase in symptom labeling, which may lead patients to overestimate the severity of his or her symptoms.

The study by Main et al. (2003) is important because the mood people are in can relate to their interpretation of symptoms. If patients with asthma have negative affect because of lower self-esteem, they may misinterpret symptoms and believe they are more symptomatic than they are. Perceptions of severity and well-being with chronic illness may have a relationship with mood and affect.

The literature has shown that chronic physical illness may impact one's self-esteem and social relationships (Bishop, 2005; Ireys et al., 1994; Livneh & Antonak, 2005, Meijer et al., 2000, Walsh & Walsh, 1987). Medication and potential side effects may also influence one's self-esteem (Carrick et al., 2004; Fornari et al., 2001; Martinez et al., 2005). Many studies only examine social support or self-esteem of one condition, such as arthritis (Abraido-Lanza, 2004, Bediako & Friend, 2004). The current study broadened the literature by examining a different construct, the relationship of a specific medication regimen. The key construct of the current study was a specific medication, not illness. Previous studies have focused on specific illness and the current study examined a specific medication.

The current study evaluated people with a chronic illness who are also currently taking prednisone. Prednisone is a common medication prescribed to control many chronic illnesses and can result in various physical side effects. The current study evaluated if taking prednisone is related to one's self-esteem and one's satisfaction with socially intimate relationships. The current study predicted that prednisone use will correlate with lower self-esteem, less satisfying socially intimate relationships and more illness intrusion.

Hypotheses

Hypothesis 1

Participants with a chronic illness who are currently taking prednisone will have lower self-esteem than those participants who are chronically ill and who have not taken prednisone in the last year. Self-esteem will be measured using the Rosenberg Self-Esteem Scale (Rosenberg, 1989).

Hypothesis 2

Participants with a chronic illness who are currently taking prednisone will have less satisfying socially intimate relationships than those participants with a chronic illness who have not taken prednisone in the last year. Social intimacy will be measured using the Miller Social Intimacy Scale (Miller & Lefcourt, 1982).

Hypothesis 3

The relationship between specific side effects and self-esteem will be examined for the prednisone group. It is predicted that there will be a negative correlation between side effects and self-esteem. Side effects are operationalized by a list of side effects which will be provided in the demographics section. Side effects will be scored using the number of side effects endorsed and the average severity of the side effects. Self-esteem will be assessed using the Rosenberg Self-Esteem Scale (Rosenberg, 1989).

Hypothesis 4

An analysis on the relationship between side effects and social intimacy will be conducted for the prednisone group. There is expected to be a negative correlation between side effects and social intimacy. Side effects are operationalized by a list of common side effects from prednisone which will be provided in the demographics section. Side effects will be scored using the number of side effects endorsed and the average severity of the side effects. Social intimacy will be measured using the Miller Social Intimacy Scale (Miller & Lefcourt, 1982).

Hypothesis 5

Female participants who use prednisone will have lower self-esteem than males who use prednisone and males and females who have not used prednisone in the past year. According to Covino et al. (1982), women with a chronic illness had more problems with self-esteem than men with a chronic illness. Self-esteem will be assessed using the Rosenberg Self-Esteem Scale (Rosenberg, 1989).

Hypothesis 6

Participants under age 50 who take prednisone will experience lower self-esteem and lower social intimacy than those participants who take prednisone and are over 50 years of age. Younger adults may hold higher expectations concerning their physical functioning than older adults (Bloom et al., 1998). Illness has been shown to be more distressing to younger individuals than older ones (Coyne & Smith, 1991). Self-esteem will be assessed using the Rosenberg Self-Esteem Scale (Rosenberg, 1989). Miller Social Intimacy Scale (Miller & Lefcourt, 1982) will be used to assess social intimacy.

Hypothesis 7

Illness intrusion will be positively correlated with side effect severity for the prednisone group. Illness intrusion will be evaluated using the Adapted Illness Intrusiveness Ratings (Stanford Research Center, 2001).

Definition of Terms

Chronic illness- An illness, in which, many times there is no cure (Covino, Dirks, Kinsman, & Seidel, 1982). Chronic illnesses develop and continue over time or reoccur over a long period of time (Brannon & Feist, 2004). About 54 million Americans suffer from a chronic illness and eight out of ten most common causes of death are a result of a chronic illness (Liveneh & Antonak, 2005). The onset of chronic illness can be a disease process, congenital, or acquired later in life (Liveneh & Antonak, 2005). People with chronic illnesses suffer from increased stress, stigma, loss, and unpredictability of an illness (Liveneh & Antonak, 2005). The diagnosis of a chronic illness results in a life-long struggle with changes in environment, social, psychological and physical abilities (Bishop, 2005). Chronic illnesses include multiple sclerosis, cancer, asthma, diabetes,

COPD, Parkinson's disease, and rheumatoid arthritis (Livneh & Antonak, 2005, Naude & Pretorius, 2003, Trief, et al. 2004).

Illness intrusion- Illness intrusiveness measures the way illness disrupts lifestyle, activities, well-being and quality of life. Illness intrusiveness refers to not only the interference of a disease but also the impact of treatment (Devins et al., 2001). Illness intrusion looks at the impact of illness on physical well-being, work and finances, social relations, sexual and family relations (Devins et al., 2001).

Illness uncertainty- Illness uncertainty is defined as the unpredictability of one's illness, treatment and prognosis (Mishel & Braden, 1988). Illness uncertainty includes lack of information and cure for one's illness (Mishel & Braden, 1998).

Prednisone- A steroid known as a glucocorticoid or corticosteroid. Prednisone resembles the natural cortical hormone produced by the adrenal glands. Prednisone is a common anti-inflammatory drug used to treat chronic inflammation illnesses (Kalibjian, 2003).

Self-esteem- Self-esteem is conceptualized as positive or negative feelings about one's self (Silver et al., 1995). Self-esteem is thought of as respect and acceptance for oneself and may have an impact on affect (Silver et al., 1995).

Social intimacy- Intimacy in various interpersonal relationships, not limited to only romantic relationships (Miller & Lefcourt, 1982). Social intimacy refers to any close relationship, either a friendship or an intimate relationship (Miller & Lefcourt, 1982). Close relationships are evaluated by frequency of contact and intensity of closeness (Miller & Lefcourt, 1982).

CHAPTER 3

Methods

Participants

Participants were adults, ages 18 and over, who have been diagnosed with a chronic physical illness. Of the 140 surveys submitted, 101 were analyzed for the study. Thirty-nine of the surveys were disqualified for incomplete data. The study resulted in 41 participants in the prednisone group and 60 participants in the non-prednisone group. Participants in the prednisone group were required to be currently taking prednisone for management of a chronic illness. Participants in the no prednisone group are required to not be currently taking prednisone. Twenty-two percent of the participants were men, and 78% of the participants were women. Eighty-six percent of the participants were Caucasian, two percent were Asian, three percent were Latino, three percent were African-American, five percent were Multiethnic and one percent was Other. The mean age of the participants was 32.2 years ($SD = 11.5$ years), with a minimum of 18 and a maximum of 62 years. Twenty-six percent of the participants were single and not dating, 22% were single and dating, 47% of the participants were married or in a committed relationship, three percent were divorced and two percent were widowed. Demographics information are presented in Table 1. Of the participants in the prednisone group, the mean length of time on prednisone was 2 years ($SD = 3.4$ years). Participants were able to read and understand English as the measures being administered have only been normed in English.

An ad was placed on craigslist.org to recruit participants. Craigslist.org is a search engine providing information for people about various opportunities including

Table 1
Demographic frequencies of Variables

	mean	median	S.D.	Minimum	Maximum
Age					
Full Sample	32	28	11.5	18	62
Prednisone Only	33.6	30	11.7	18	62
Non-Prednisone	31.28	28	11.5	18	62
Income					
Full Sample	35099.01	30000	38,000.39	3000	200000
Prednisone Only	53606.06	30000	42778.45	6000	200000
Non-Prednisone	42285.71	16000	31367.44	3000	130000

Varible	Percent	n	Prednisone Percent	n	Non-Prednisone Percent	N
Gender						
male	22	22	19.5	8	21.7	13
female	78	79	80.5	33	78.3	47
Ethnicity						
Caucasian	87	88	82.9	34	88.3	53
Latino	3	3	4.8	2	1.7	1
African-American	2	2	2.5	1	3.3	2
Asian American	2	2	2.5	1	1.7	1
Multi-Ethnic	5	5	4.8	2	5	3
Other	1	1	2.5	1	0	0
Education						
some high school	3	3	7.4	3	0	0
high school graduate	4	4	2.5	1	5	3
some college	33	33	29.2	12	35	21
college graduate	35	35	26.8	11	40	24
some grad school	12	12	12.2	5	11.7	7
grad school degree	14	14	21.9	9	8.3	5
Marital Status						
single, not dating	26	26	31.7	13	21.7	0
single, dating	22	22	19.6	8	23.3	3
married	29.7	30	31.7	13	28.3	21
commited relationship	17.80	18	9.7	4	23.3	23
divorced	3	3	4.8	2	1.7	7
widowed	2	2	2.5	1	1.7	5

Table 1 continued

Employment						
student	33	33	24.4	10	38.4	23
part time	11	11	7.3	3	13.3	8
full time	33	33	36.6	15	30	18
unemployment	4	4	4.9	2	3.3	2
disability	20	20	26.8	11	15	9

employment, housing and even volunteer opportunities. Advertisements were placed on various chronic illness chat rooms including www.healingwell.com, http://p208.ezboard.com/fbeentheredonethatfrm1, http://messageboards.ivillage.com, www.butyoudontlooksick.com/boards, www.thelupuslady.com, and http://health.yahoo.com/groups.

Measures

Demographics Questionnaire

Participants filled out a demographic questionnaire assessing age, gender, education, income, chronic illness diagnosis, and length of time since diagnosis. Participants were asked if they have ever taken a medication for longer than 3 months, if they are currently on any medication, if they have ever taken prednisone, length of treatment, dose, and how long ago the medication was taken. Participants who have taken medication were asked to identify the side effects they experienced from a list of side effects and complete a side effects severity rating. Participants were asked to complete the questionnaire based on the medication they are currently taking or have taken most recently. The list of side effects was complied from a list of prednisone side effects as well as side effects from other medications. Medication side effects were obtained from www.drugs.com. Side effects that were congruent with symptoms of illness were omitted from the list.

Rosenberg Self-Esteem Scale (Rosenberg, 1989)

The Rosenberg Self-Esteem Scale (RSES) measures one's feelings towards oneself and one's value. Self-esteem is one component of self-concept. The scale was originally developed in the 1960s and was administered to 5,024 juniors and seniors at ten different New York high schools. The scale is reliable with a test-retest score of .82 to .88 and Cronbach's alpha of .77 to .88. Whiteside-Mansell and Corwyn (2003) have found that the Rosenberg Self-Esteem Scale yielded comparable results for adolescents and adults. The follow-up analysis also indicted there were no mean differences between the two groups (Whiteside-Mansell & Corwyn, 2003). Concurrent correlations ranging from .72 to .76 were found between the Rosenberg Self-Esteem Scale and the Single Item Self-Esteem Scale demonstrating construct validity (Robins, Hendin & Trzesniewski, 2001). The Rosenberg Self-Esteem was strongly related to the Self-Perception Profile sub-index evaluating global self-worth which supports that the RSES is evaluating self-esteem (Hagborg, 1993).

The Rosenberg Self-Esteem Scale consists of ten items rated on a Likert scale from one (strongly agree) to five (strongly disagree). Items three, five, eight, nine and ten are reversed scored. The numbers are then added up to receive a total score. A low score reflects high self-esteem and a high score reflects low self-esteem. Two example items are "I feel that I'm a person of worth, at least on an equal plane with others" and "I take a positive attitude toward myself" (Rosenberg, 1989).

Miller Social Intimacy Scale (Miller & Lefcourt, 1982)

The Miller Social Intimacy Scale (MSIS) assesses intimacy in a romantic relationship or a friendship. Even though the scale is 25 years old, the Miller Social Intimacy Scale was chosen because it was applicable to not only romantic relationships but friendships as well. The scale contains 17 items, six evaluating frequency of interactions and 11 examining the intensity of these interactions on a 10 point Likert scale. Questions are rated on a Likert scale for frequency ratings ranged from "1" very rarely to "10" almost always. The intensity ratings ranged from "1" meaning not much to "10" meaning a great deal. Items two and 14 are reverse scored. Participants complete the survey in regards to their spouse or closest friendship. A sample item examining intensity of the interaction is "How important is it to you that he/she be encouraging and supportive when you are unhappy?" A sample of the frequency of interactions is "How often do you confide very personal information to him/her?" (Miller & Lefcourt, 1982).

The Miller Social Intimacy Scale has a Cronbach's alpha of .91. The scale also had $r=.96$ test-retest reliability over two months and $r=.84$ test-retest reliability over one month, demonstrating relative stability over time. The mean of the MSIS scores were higher for descriptions of close friends compared to casual friends. The mean MSIS score was significantly greater for married participants than unmarried participants($t=8.17$, n=25), which supports the construct that marital relationships result in greater intimacy than non-married couples (Miller & Lefcourt, 1982). Participants who rated themselves as lonely on the UCLA Loneliness Scale scored low on the Miller Social Intimacy Scale($r=-.65$).

Adapted Illness Intrusiveness Ratings developed by Stanford Research Center (2001)

The Adapted Illness Intrusiveness Rating was based on the Illness Intrusiveness Rating developed by Devins et al. (1983). The adapted version of the scale was changed so the wording was more clear and easier to understand. The 13 item scale measures how much illness and treatment interferes with life. Questions included "How much does your illness interfere with your feelings of being healthy?" "How much does your illness affect the things you eat and drink?" "How much does your illness affect your relationship with spouse or domestic partner?" Questions are rated on a Likert scale ranging from (1) "not very much" to (7) "very much". The Adapted Illness Intrusiveness Rating has an internal consistency reliability of .89. No information was reported regarding the validity of the measure. The scale was given to 606 participants with chronic illnesses. The original Illness Intrusion Scale (Devins et al., 1983) was administered to 70 participants with end-stage renal disease (ESRD). Greater illness intrusion was associated with lower perceived control over dialysis ($r=-.25$) and ESRD ($r=-.41$), higher ratings of illness intrusion by hospital staff ($r=.36$) and significant others ($r=.26$) (Devins, et al. 1983). High levels of illness intrusion were significantly correlated with decreased positive mood and increased negative mood (Devins, et al., 1983).

Procedures

Participants were recruited from Internet advertisements on craigslist.org and from chat rooms at www.healingwell.com, www.butyoudontlooksick.com/boards, http://p208.ezboard.com/fbeentheredonethatfrm1, http://messageboards.ivillage.com, , www.thelupuslady.com, and http://health.yahoo.com/groups. Internet advertisements directed participants to a surveymonkey.com account where they completed the surveys. Surveymonkey.com is a secure website for data collection. After clicking on the link, participants were brought to the surveymonkey.com site that first provided a welcome letter explaining the study and requirements for participation. Then participants were directed to an informed consent page which gave further detail about the study and informed the participant that the study was voluntary and provided the email address of the researcher in case they had further questions or concerns. Participants were provided with the option of receiving a summary of the study results. In order to receive the results, participants checked a box and provided an address for the results to be delivered. Participants then checked a box agreeing to participate in the study. Once agreeing to participate, participants completed the demographic questionnaires, Rosenberg Self-Esteem Scale (Rosenberg, 1989), Miller Social Intimacy Scale (Miller & Lefcourt, 1982), and Adapted Illness Intrusiveness Ratings (Stanford Research Center, 2001). Participants answered each question before moving on to the next page. Once they finished the scales, participants clicked submit in order to submit the completed scales to the researcher. Finally the participants were directed to a letter thanking them for their participation. After completion of the study, the data will be kept for five years in a locked file cabinet at the researcher's home office. After five years, the questionnaires and consent forms will be shredded by the researcher.

Design

The current study is a between subjects two group (prednisone use and no prednisone) non-experimental design examining self-esteem, social intimacy, and illness intrusion among people with chronic illness who have and have not taken prednisone. . The independent variable in this study is prednisone use. The dependent variables were self-esteem (measured by the Rosenberg Self-Esteem Scale), social intimacy (measured by the Miller Social Intimacy Scale) and illness intrusion (Adapted Illness Intrusiveness Rating).

CHAPTER 4

Results

Means and standard deviations for age of diagnosis of a chronic illness, age of first medication prescribed, and number of medications taken were provided for all participants. Medical information is presented in Table 2. Frequencies of each medication taken were reported. The average side effects intensity was also be reported. All of the side effects ratings ranged between zero to five.

<u>Demographic and Study Variables</u>

The data were normally distributed and there were no outliers more than three standard deviations from the mean. Thirty-nine of the original 140 surveys were disqualified for failure to complete the survey questions. Relationships between the study variables and demographics were examined. Demographics that are related to the dependent variables were covaried out of the correlational analysis. Self-esteem was significantly related to education, the more education received, the higher the reported self-esteem. Younger people reported greater intimacy in their intimate relationships than older participants. Social intimacy was significantly related to income, the lower the income, the greater the level of reported social intimacy. Illness intrusion was significantly related to age, the older the participant, the more illness intrusion experienced. Illness intrusion was significantly related to gender. An independent t-test was conducted to compare gender with self-esteem, social intimacy and illness intrusion. Gender was significantly related to illness intrusion, $t(99)=-2.22, p=.008$. Females reported experiencing more illness intrusion than male participants. Gender was not significantly related to social intimacy, $t(99)=-2.469, p=.063$ or self-esteem, $t(99)=.572$,

Table 2
Medical Information for Participants

Full Sample	Mean	Median	S.D.	Minimum	Maximum
Age of Diagnosis	22	20	11.5	0	61
Length of Diagnosis (in years)	9.5	6	8.9	0.08	36
Years currently taking Prednisone	2	0.05	3.4	0	16
Number of Different Medications Taken	5.2	4	5.5	0	30
Age first given medication	21.7	20	12.4	0	62

Prednisone Group Only	Mean	Median	S.D.	Minimum	Maximum
Age of Diagnosis	22.85	20	12.16	0	60
Length of Diagnosis (in years)	9.26	5	9.37	0.08	36
Years currently taking Prednisone	2	0.05	3.4	0	16
Number of Different Medications Taken	6	4	7.07	0	30
Age first given medication	22.17	20	11.73	0	60

Not Currently Taking Prednisone Group	Mean	Median	S.D.	Minimum	Maximum
Age of Diagnosis	21.45	20	12.74	1	61
Length of diagnosis (in years)	9.76	7	8.68	0.25	35
Number of Different Medications Taken	4.68	4	4.11	0	20
Age first given medication	21.53	20	12.86	1	62

Diagnosis-Full Sample	n	Percentage
Asthma	31	30.70%
Crohn's Disease	28	27.70%
Ulcerative Colitis	8	7.90%
RA	7	6.90%
Diabetes	4	4%
Cancer	1	1%
HIV	1	1%
Other	21	20.80%

Table 2 continued

Diagnosis-Prednisone Group Only	n	Percentage
Asthma	16	39
Crohn's Disease	5	12.2
Ulcerative Colitis	5	12.2
RA	3	7.3
Diabetes	2	4.9
Cancer	0	0
HIV	0	0
Other	10	24.4

Diagnosis-Not Currently Taking Prednisone	n	Percentage
Asthma	14	23.3
Crohn's Disease	24	40
Ulcerative Colitis	3	5
RA	4	6.7
Diabetes	2	3.3
Cancer	1	1.7
HIV	1	1.7
Other	11	18.3

$p=.249$. A one-way ANOVA was conducted and ethnicity was not significantly correlated with self-esteem $F(5,95)=.28, p=.921$, social intimacy $F(5,95)=1.8, p=.12$, or illness intrusion $F(5,95)=1.91, p=.099$. A one way ANOVA was conducted examining ethnicity split into participants that are Caucasian (n=87) and not Caucasian (n=14). When ethnicity was split in this way, ethnicity was not significantly related to self-esteem $F(1,99)=.196, p=.659$ or social intimacy $F(1,99)=1.476, p=.227$. Illness intrusion was significantly related to ethnicity $F(1,99)=8.26, p=.005$ when ethnicity was divided into participants that are Caucasian (n=87) and not Caucasian (n=14). Few studies have examined the relationship between specific side effects related to self-esteem, social intimacy and illness intrusion.

Due to the number of correlations conducted in this exploratory examination, a Bonferroni correction was conducted. With the stringency of the Bonferroni correction, few results reached statistical significance. However, because of the exploratory nature of this investigation and the relatively innovative examination of side effects, results presented at the .05 significant level suggest relationships warranting further study. Correlation coefficients are reported in Table 3.

<u>Correlation of Study Variables</u>

Pearson's correlations were conducted to assess relationships among study variables. Self-esteem and social intimacy were significantly correlated, $r=-.218, p=.029$. Self-esteem and illness intrusion were significantly correlated, $r=.211, p=.034$. Social intimacy and illness intrusion were significantly correlated, $r=-.380, p<.000$.

Table 3
Correlation of Demographic and Study Variables

Study Variable	Demographic Variables		
	age	income	education
Self-Esteem	-0.116	-0.128	-0.25*
Social Intimacy	-0.207*	-0.266**	0.077
Illness Intrusion	0.251*	0.173	-0.006

* Correlation significant at the 0.05 level
** Correlation significant at the 0.01 level

Comparison of Prednisone Group and Control Group

When comparing the prednisone and control group, they did not differ significantly on demographic variables, including education level, age, gender, or income. Therefore, demographic variables were not considered in analyses of hypotheses comparing the two groups.

Hypotheses

Hypothesis 1

An independent t test was conducted to compare if participants with a chronic illness who are currently taking prednisone reported lower self-esteem than those participants who are chronically ill and who are not currently taking prednisone. Self-esteem was measured using the Rosenberg Self-Esteem Scale (Rosenberg, 1989). The prednisone group was not significantly different than the non prednisone control group, $t(99)= -.728$, $p=.958$. The mean for the prednisone group was 24.61 and the standard deviation was 9.15 and the effect size was -.147. The mean for the group not currently taking prednisone was 25.96 and the standard deviation was 9.23.

Hypothesis 2

An independent t test was conducted to see if participants with a chronic illness who are currently on prednisone report less intimate relationships than those participants with a chronic illness who are not currently taking prednisone. Social intimacy was measured using the Miller Social Intimacy Scale (Miller & Lefcourt, 1982). The prednisone group was not significantly different than the control group, $t(99)= -1.88$, $p=.158$. The mean for the prednisone group was 120.78 and the standard deviation was

27.46 and the effect size was -.380. The mean for the group not currently taking prednisone was 130.50 and the standard deviation was 24.11.

Hypothesis 3A

A Pearson's correlation was conducted to examine the relationship between specific side effects and self-esteem for the prednisone group (n=41). Side effects were rated based on severity on a five point Likert Scale. Each side effect severity rating for each individual side effect was correlated separately with self-esteem. Self-esteem was assessed using the Rosenberg Self-Esteem Scale (Rosenberg, 1989). Self-esteem was significant negative correlation at the .05 significance level with mood swings, acne, unusual tiredness, and headaches. Self-esteem was significantly negatively correlated at the .01 significance level with sexual side effects and dizziness. See Table 4 for correlation coefficients. When a partial correlation was done controlling for education level, self-esteem was still significantly negatively related to sexual side effects and dizziness at the .01 level and mood swings at the .05 level. The relationship with acne and unusual tiredness was no longer significant. In general, the pattern of the relationship was the same for both the correlation and the partial correlation.

Hypothesis 3B

A Pearson's correlation was conducted to examine the relationship between specific side effects and self-esteem for all participants that currently reported being on any medication (n=93). Side effects were rated based on severity on a five point Likert Scale. Each side effect severity rating for each individual side effect was correlated separately with self- esteem. Self-esteem was assessed using the Rosenberg Self-Esteem Scale (Rosenberg, 1989). Self-esteem was significantly negatively correlated at the .05

Table 4
Pearson's Correlation Matrix of Side Effects and Self-Esteem, Social Intimacy and Illness Intrusion for the Prednisone Group Only

Side Effects	Self-Esteem	Significant	Social Intimacy	Significant	Illness Intrusion	Significant
rounding of face	0.240	0.131	0.098	0.542	0.417**	0.007
stretch marks	0.065	0.686	-0.180	0.261	0.493**	0.001
weight gain	0.094	0.561	-0.120	0.938	0.396**	0.010
hair loss	0.096	0.550	-0.990	0.539	0.302*	0.055
facial hair	0.209	0.190	-0.227	0.153	0.425**	0.006
mood swings	0.304*	0.053	-0.258	0.104	0.523**	0.000
acne	0.270*	0.088	-0.247	0.119	0.366**	0.019
unusual tiredness	0.284*	0.072	-0.266*	0.092	0.597**	0.000
nausea	0.160	0.319	-0.700	0.664	0.253	0.111
difficulty sleeping	0.197	0.321	-0.137	0.394	0.613**	0.000
dry mouth	0.116	0.472	-0.317*	0.044	0.517**	0.001
headache	0.289*	0.067	-0.206	0.196	0.286*	0.070
sexual side effects	0.377**	0.015	-0.393**	0.011	0.418**	0.007
dizziness	0.469**	0.002	-0.001	0.993	0.400**	0.010

** Correlation significant < 0.01 level
* Correlation significant < 0.05 level

*Note: Rosenberg Self-Esteem Scale is inverse scored, such that high scores reflect lower self-esteem.

level with nausea and dizziness. See Table 5 for correlation coefficients. When a partial correlation was done controlling for education, the pattern of the relationship was the same for both the correlation and the partial correlation. The partial correlation resulted in strengthening the relationship between self-esteem and dizziness at the .01 level and nausea remained the same being significant at the .05 level.

Hypothesis 4A

A Pearson's correlation was conducted to examine the relationship between specific side effects and satisfying socially intimate relationships for the prednisone group (n=41). Social intimacy was measured using the Miller Social Intimacy Scale (Miller & Lefcourt, 1982). Side effects were rated based on severity on five point Likert Scale. Each side effect severity rating for each individual side effect was correlated separately with social intimacy. Social intimacy was significantly negatively correlated at the .05 level with unusual tiredness and dry mouth. Social intimacy was significantly negatively correlated at the .01 level with sexual side effects. See Table 4 for the correlation coefficients. When a partial correlation was done controlling for age and income, the relationship between social intimacy and sexual side effects and dry mouth remained significant. The significant relationship between social intimacy and unusual tiredness was lost when a partial correlation was done.

Hypothesis 4B

A Pearson's correlation was conducted to examine the relationship between specific side effects and satisfying socially intimate relationships for all participants that currently reported being on any medication (n=93). Social intimacy was measured using

Table 5

Pearson's Correlation Matrix of Side Effects and Self-Esteem, Social Intimacy and Illness Intrusion For the prednisone and control groups

Side Effects	Self-Esteem	Significant	Social Intimacy	Significant	Illness Intrusion	Significant
rounding of face	0.118	0.259	-0.034	0.750	0.351**	0.001
stretch marks	0.001	0.993	-0.137	0.190	0.321**	0.002
weight gain	0.054	0.607	-0.077	0.463	0.390**	0.000
hair loss	-0.025	0.812	-0.010	0.923	0.319**	0.002
facial hair	0.005	0.962	-0.027	0.797	0.282**	0.006
mood swings	0.136	0.194	-0.240*	0.020	0.473**	0.000
acne	0.100	0.340	-0.109	0.300	0.232*	0.025
unusual tiredness	0.091	0.387	-0.205*	0.049	0.508**	0.000
nausea	0.209*	0.044	-0.058	0.579	0.312**	0.002
difficulty sleeping	0.155	0.137	-0.202*	0.052	0.583**	0.000
dry mouth	0.143	0.171	-0.258**	0.013	0.451**	0.000
headache	0.145	0.164	-0.059	0.577	0.386**	0.000
sexual side effects	0.134	0.199	-0.016	0.119	0.302**	0.003
dizziness	0.265*	0.013	-0.016	0.878	0.399**	0.000

** Correlation significant < 0.01 level
* Correlation significant < 0.05 level

*Note: Rosenberg Self-Esteem Scale is inverse scored, such that high scores reflect lower self-esteem.

the Miller Social Intimacy Scale (Miller & Lefcourt, 1982). Side effects were rated based on severity on five point Likert Scale. Each side effect severity rating for each individual side effect was correlated separately with social intimacy. Social intimacy was significantly negatively correlated at the .05 level with unusual tiredness, dry mouth, and mood swings. See Table 5 for the correlation coefficients. When a partial correlation was done controlling for age and income, the relationship between social intimacy and mood swings, unusual tiredness and dry mouth was strengthened and a significant negative correlation between social intimacy and trouble sleeping emerged at the .05 level.

Hypothesis 5

A 2 way ANOVA was conducted to see if female participants who are currently taking prednisone have lower self-esteem than males and females who are not currently taking prednisone. Self-esteem was measured using the Rosenberg Self-Esteem Scale (Rosenberg, 1989). Gender was not statistically significant $F(1, 97)=.55, p=.46$. Prednisone was not statistically significant $F(1, 97)=.003, p=.956$. The interaction effect was not statistically significant $F(1, 97)=.782, p=.379$ and the effect size was .008.

Hypothesis 6A

An independent *t* test was conducted to compare if participants who take prednisone and under 50 (n=34) experience lower self-esteem than those participants who take prednisone and 50 and over (n=6). One participant did not report their age. The Rosenberg Self-Esteem Scale (Rosenberg, 1989) was used to measure self-esteem. Participants under 50 who are taking prednisone did not experience significantly lower self-esteem, t(38)=.836, p=.180, effect size .163, when compared to participants 50 and over currently taking prednisone.

Hypothesis 6B

An independent t test was conducted to compare if participants who take prednisone and under 50 (n=34) lower social intimacy than those participants who take prednisone and 50 and over (n=6). One participant did not report their age. Social intimacy was assessed using the Miller Social Intimacy Scale (Miller & Lefcourt, 1982). Participants under 50 who are taking prednisone did not experience significantly lower social intimacy, t(38)= .628, p=.256, effect size .123, when compared to participants 50 and over currently taking prednisone.

Hypothesis 6C

An independent t test was conducted to compare if participants under 50 (n=88) experience lower self-esteem than those participants 50 and over (n=12). One participant did not report their age. The Rosenberg Self-Esteem Scale (Rosenberg, 1989) was used to measure self-esteem. Participants under 50 who are taking prednisone did not experience significantly lower self-esteem, t(98)= .602, p=.440, effect size .185, when compared to participants 50 and over currently taking prednisone.

Hypothesis 6D

An independent t test was conducted to compare if participants under 50 (n=88) reported lower social intimacy than those participants 50 and over (n=12). One participant did not report their age. Social intimacy was assessed using the Miller Social Intimacy Scale (Miller & Lefcourt, 1982). Participants under 50 who are taking prednisone did not experience significantly lower social intimacy, $t(98)= .186, p=.668$, effect size .0572, when compared to participants 50 and over currently taking prednisone.

Hypothesis 7A

A Pearson's correlation was conducted to compare if side effect severity is correlated with illness intrusion for the prednisone group (n=41). Each side effect severity rating for each individual side effect was correlated separately with illness intrusion. Illness intrusion was evaluated using the Adapted Illness Intrusiveness Ratings (Stanford Research Center, 2001). Illness intrusion was significantly positively correlated at the .05 level with headaches and hair loss. Illness intrusion was significantly positively correlated at the .01 level with rounding of the face, stretch marks, weight gain, increased facial hair, mood swings, acne unusual tiredness, difficulty sleeping, dry mouth, sexual side effects and dizziness. See Table 4 for correlation coefficients. When a partial correlation was done controlling for age and gender, the general pattern of relationships was the same. The relationship between illness intrusion and headaches lost significance when controlling for age and gender. A linear regression was conducted to control for ethnicity, the general pattern of relationships remained the same. Hair loss and headaches both lost significance when controlling for ethnicity. The strength of the relationship between acne and illness intrusion reduced to the .05 level and a relationship between nausea and illness intrusion was found at the .05 level.

Hypothesis 7B

A Pearson's correlation was conducted to compare if side effect severity is correlated with illness intrusion for all participants that currently reported being on medication (n=93). Each side effect severity rating for each individual side effect was correlated separately with self-esteem. Illness intrusion was evaluated using the Adapted Illness Intrusiveness Ratings (Stanford Research Center, 2001). Illness intrusion was significantly positively correlated at the .05 level with acne. Illness intrusion was significantly positively correlated at the .01 level with rounding of the face, stretch marks weight gain, hair loss, increased facial hair, mood swings, unusual tiredness, nausea, difficulty sleeping, dry mouth, headaches, sexual side effects and dizziness. See Table 5 for correlation coefficients. When a partial correlation was done controlling for age and gender, the pattern of the relationship remained the same. The relationship between illness intrusion and acne was strengthened when controlling for age and gender. A linear regression was conducted to control for ethnicity, the general pattern of relationships remained the same.

Bonferroni Correction

A Bonferroni Correction was conducted for Hypotheses 3A, 3B, 4A, 4B, 7A and 7B. Using a Bonferroni adjusted alpha level of 0.0035, the relationship between self-esteem, social intimacy and specific side effects was no longer significant. Using a Bonferroni adjusted alpha level of 0.0035, illness intrusion in participants currently using prednisone was significantly positively correlated with stretch marks, mood swings, unusual tiredness, difficulty sleeping, and dry mouth at the .05 level. Using a Bonferroni adjusted alpha level of 0.0035, illness intrusion in all participants currently using medication was significantly positively correlated with rounding of the face, stretch marks, weight gain, hair loss, mood swings, unusual tiredness, nausea, difficulty sleeping, dry mouth, headache, sexual side effects, and dizziness at the .05 level.

Post Hoc Analysis

A post hoc analysis was conducted using an independent t-test to compare if participants with a chronic illness who are currently taking prednisone reported higher severity of side effects than participants who are chronically ill and are not currently taking prednisone. The prednisone group reported significantly higher ratings on four side effects; stretch marks, $t=3.64$, $p<.000$, hair loss, $t=1.868$, $p=.019$, acne, $t=1.929$, $p=.02$, and dry mouth, $t=2.723$, $p<.000$. There was no other statistically significant difference between the groups.

CHAPTER 5

Discussion

Medications used to treat chronic illness have potential side effects that may intensify the impact of chronic illness on body image, self-esteem and well being(Carrick, et al., 2004; Fornari, et al., 2001; Martinez, et al., 2005). For instance, negative body image was correlated with symptoms, either due to chronic illness or medication side effects (Martinez, et al., 2005).

Medications can result in a variety of physical side effects. Prednisone is a widely used medication in the treatment of inflammatory illnesses in children and adults. Prednisone is a steroid and can result in an array of physical and emotional side effects such as facial swelling, facial and body hair growth, stretch marks, mood swings, insomnia, acne, hair loss and weight gain (Kalibjian, 2003; Skylar, 2002). Due to the rapid changes in one's appearance, the current study examined the impact of the side effects of these medications on self-esteem and social intimacy. Covino et al. (1982) found that patients with asthma had the lowest self-esteem when compared to patients with pain or tuberculosis. The study by Covino et al. (1982) did not indicate why there was a difference in self-esteem between the three groups, but perhaps it was due to the difference in medication treatment and associated side effects. Prednisone is commonly used to treat asthma, and associated side effects may contribute to the difference Covino et al. (1982) found. There has been little research looking at the relationship between prednisone use and self-esteem and social intimacy in a chronically ill population.

Prednisone may be some patients' only treatment option for their condition (Skylar, 2002). Due to the unpleasant side effects, patients may adapt coping strategies to deal with prednisone side effects, such as controlling diet, exercise and skin care. The current study was conducted with the goal of providing valuable information for mental health professionals and physicians treating patients taking prednisone.

The current study examined the relationship between prednisone use and self-esteem, social intimacy, and illness intrusion in a chronically ill population. Self-esteem is conceptualized as positive or negative feelings about one's self (Silver et al., 1995). There is very little literature available about the impact of prednisone use on self-esteem, social intimacy and illness intrusion. In one study, participants with MS reported lower levels of self-esteem, lower levels of seeking social support and higher levels of detachment when compared to the general population (McCabe & Di Battista, 2004). Prednisone is used in the treatment of MS which may have contributed to some of the results in the study by McCabe and Di Battista (2004). Prednisone had been linked to various disorders. For example, Fornari et al. (2001) found that 2% of people who presented in the eating disorder clinic were prescribed a steroid shortly before the onset of the eating disorder. Taking medications, such as prednisone, can have an impact on one's life. Medication side effects can be disruptive to a person's life as found in a study by Carrick et al. (2004). The current study sought to expand the literature and provide information about prednisone use and its relationship to self-esteem, social intimacy and illness intrusion.

No differences were found across any of the three study variables (self-esteem, social intimacy and illness intrusion) when comparing individuals with a chronic illness who used prednisone compared with individuals with a chronic illness who were not currently using prednisone. The four side effects that significantly differed in reported severity for the prednisone and group not currently taking prednisone were not side effects that were significantly correlated with self-esteem, social intimacy and illness intrusion. The side effects significantly related to self-esteem, social intimacy and illness intrusion are stretch marks, hair loss, acne and dry mouth. The side effects that appeared to consistently relate to self-esteem, social intimacy and illness intrusion were experienced similarly by both the prednisone group and group not currently taking prednisone.

Side effects were then correlated with self-esteem, social intimacy and illness intrusion for all participants currently on medication in both the prednisone and control group. Unusual tiredness and sexual side effects were significantly negatively correlated to self-esteem across all those with a chronic illness who were currently taking medication. Social intimacy was significantly negatively correlated with mood swings, unusual tiredness and dry mouth for the full sample of participants with a chronic illness. Illness intrusion was significantly positively related to severity of side effects across 13 of the 15 side effects endorsed. Results suggest that experiencing side effects has a relationship with self-esteem, social intimacy and illness intrusion, regardless of what medication produces the side effects.

Because of the correlational nature of the study, directionality of results can not be determined. This study has found that severity of side effects may impact one's self-esteem, social intimacy and illness intrusion, regardless of the medication that produces the side effects. Taking a medication that results in physical changes may relate to one's self-esteem, social intimacy and illness intrusion. Experiencing physical side effects may impact the way one view's themselves, which may relate to one's self-esteem. The experience of having side effects may lead to a patient withdrawing, which would impact their social intimacy. A patient may have an increase in illness intrusion due to the side effects he or she is experiencing. Results may also support that people with lower self-esteem, social intimacy and who experience more illness intrusion have a tendency to report experiencing more side effects or are more sensitive to the experience of having side effects. Participants with lower self-esteem prior to beginning prednisone treatment may have magnified minor changes in their physical appearance, resulting in higher ratings of side effect severity. Participants with high self-esteem prior to beginning prednisone treatment may not have been bothered by physical changes and therefore reported lower side effect severity. The experience of side effects is subjective, therefore it is a complicated process to compare individuals based on subjective reports. Due to the subjective nature of side effects, it is difficult to understand directionality.

It is not necessarily taking prednisone that produces this effect, but taking any medication that produces numerous, bothersome side effects. Illness intrusion was significantly positively correlated with almost all of the side effects in the prednisone group as well as across the entire sample of individuals with chronic illness that take medications. In the prednisone group, self-esteem was significantly negatively correlated with physical side effects, such as acne as well as headache, sexual side effects, unusual tiredness and mood swings. In the prednisone group, social intimacy was significantly negatively related to dry mouth, unusual tiredness and sexual side effects.

Patterns remained consistent throughout the results when controlling for the influence of demographics. Clinicians should be aware of influences of demographic factors including education, ethnicity, gender and age as they relate to the relationship between side effects and self-esteem, social intimacy and illness intrusion.

The two groups did not differ significantly in terms of self-esteem, social intimacy and illness intrusion, which may have happened for a variety of reasons. Having a pure sample of participants who have never taken prednisone may have resulted in different results. Many of the participants in the current study had taken prednisone at some time during the course of their illness. Prednisone is the 16th most commonly prescribed medication and is used for a variety of chronic illnesses (World Almanac & Book of Facts, 2003). It is challenging to find a pure sample of people who have never used prednisone because it is so commonly prescribed. Finding a pure sample of people who have not used prednisone would be useful because the side effects of prednisone can linger after the medication is stopped. Many medications used to treat chronic illnesses may produce a similar pattern of side effects lessening the implication of prednisone, specifically. Perhaps it is the presence of side effects, regardless of the medication taken, that has a relationship with self-esteem, social intimacy and illness intrusion.

<u>Clinical Implications</u>

Patients may experience changes in self-esteem as a result of the side effects they experience. The current study was a correlational study so directionality of the changes between self-esteem and the experience of side effects cannot be determined. It may be the more side effects experienced, results in lower self-esteem. Changes in physical appearance due to side effects may result in lower self-esteem. Experiencing side effects may result in a decrease of social activities which would impact social intimacy. Illness intrusion may increase when side effects are present. Alternatively, patients with lower self-esteem may be sensitive to the side effects and reported greater severity. Participants with lower self-esteem may be more sensitive to the changes in their physical appearance, resulting in higher ratings of side effect severity. High self-esteem may serve as a protective factor and participants with high self-esteem may have reported lower side effect severity, even when side effects were present. Physicians may want to be aware of the possible impact of side effects when prescribing medications resulting in numerous of side effects. Physicians should monitor changes in the demeanor of their patient. If physicians are aware of the potential for changes in self-esteem, they can monitor these factors during exams and refer patients to therapy or groups as needed. If physicians are aware of the potential impact on self-esteem, they can be more proactive before the emotional effects become overwhelming.

Assumptions and Limitations

The current study is a correlational study and therefore causation cannot be determined. The study variables were not manipulated, therefore a correlational relationship was demonstrated. A comparison group of individuals with a chronic illness who are not currently taking prednisone were used. The current study is cross-sectional evaluating participants at one point in time. A more accurate way to evaluate individuals over time is by utilizing a longitudinal study.

Random assignment was not utilized in this study. Participants were not randomly assigned to an illness group or a medication group, consequently the groups were naturally divided based on history. Participants were recruited through chat rooms and craigslist.org hence the study results are only generalizable to those who have access to the Internet.

Participants currently not taking prednisone were not asked the length of time prednisone was taken previously. The length of time of prednisone use by participants not currently taking prednisone would have been valuable information to have. Finding a pure sample of participants that has never taken prednisone would be valuable but challenging. Future studies may receive different results than the current study if they utilize a pure sample that has never taken prednisone.

The current study utilized questionnaires that are shown to be valid as well as reliable. The questionnaires being used rely on self report. Some limitations may occur when using self report measures since the results are dependent on participants responding honestly. The experience of side effects is subjective, which complicates the interpretations of results. Conclusions were based on the assumptions that participants responded truthfully knowing that the results remained confidential.

Further Research

Further research could be done examining the impact of prednisone on self-esteem and social intimacy compared to a medication with no or few side effects. A longitudinal study looking at self-esteem, social intimacy and illness intrusion over time could help researchers understand the directional impact of prednisone use. A longitudinal study could capture if changes in self-esteem, social intimacy and illness intrusion occur over time. A longitudinal study would be able to evaluate participant's self-esteem and social intimacy before taking prednisone and while on prednisone and therefore may evaluate the actual impact of prednisone. Future research could use a repeated measures, within subjects design to evaluate participants over the course of treatment. Further research could be done looking at pure samples of people who have never taken prednisone compared to those on prednisone for a long period of time. Having participants who have never used prednisone could control for the possibility of residual side effects from prednisone. Further research could be conducted to investigate the impact of medication side effects on self-esteem, social intimacy and illness intrusion, regardless of the medication being taken. The current study showed a correlation between medication side effects and self-esteem, social intimacy and illness intrusion. There is much research that could be continued in this field and would help to enrich the medical and psychological literature.

References

Abraido-Lanza, A.F. (2004). Social support and psychological adjustment among Latinas with arthritis: a test of a theoretical model. *Annals of Behavioral Medicine, 27*(3), 162-171.

American Psychiatric Association. (2000). *Diagnostic and statistical manual of mental Disorders(text revision)*. Washington, D.C.

Badr, H. & Acitelli, L. K. (2005). Dyadic adjustment in chronic illness: does relationship talk matter? *Journal of Family Psychology, 19*(3), 465-469.

Barrera, M., Jr., Sandler, I.N., & Ramsey, T.B. (1981). Preliminary development of a scale of social support: Studies on college students. *American Journal of Community Psychology, 9,* 435-447.

Bediako, S.M. & Friend, R. (2004). Illness-specific and general perceptions of social relationships in adjustment to Rheumatoid Arthritis: the role of interpersonal expectations. *Annals of Behavioral Medicine, 28*(3), 203-210.

Berry, D.C., Michas, I.C., & Bersellini, E. (2002). Communicating information about medication side effects: effects on satisfaction, perceived risk to health, and intention to comply. *Psychology and Health, 17*(3), 247-267.

Berry, D.C., Michas, I.C., & Bersellini, E(2003). Communicating information about medication: the benefits of making it personal. *Psychology and Health. 18*(1), 127-139.

Bishop, M. (2005). Quality of life and psychosocial adaptation to chronic illness and disability: preliminary analysis of a conceptual and theoretical synthesis. *Rehabilitation Counseling Bulletin. 48*(4), 219-231.

Bloom, J. R., Stewart, S. L., Johnston, M., & Banks, P. (1998). Intrusiveness of illness and quality of life in young women with breast cancer. *Psycho-Oncology. 7,* 89-100.

Brannon, L. & Feist, J. (2004). *Health Psychology: An introduction to behavior and Health.* Belmont, CA: Wadsworth.

Carrick, R., Mitchell, A., Powell, R., & Lloyd, K. (2004). The quest for well-being: A qualitative study of the experience of taking antipsychotic medication. *Psychology and Psychotherapy: Theory, Research and Practice. 77,* 19-33.

Carter, R. & Carter, C. (1994). Martial adjustment and effects of illness in married pairs with one or both spouses chronically ill. *The American Journal of Family Therapy. 22* (4), 315-326.

Conn, V.S., Taylor, S.G., & Hayes, V. (1992). Social support, self-esteem and self-care after myocardial infarction. *The Journal of Health Behavior, Education and Promotion, 16*(5), 25-32.

Covino, N. A., Dirks, J.F., Kinsman, R.A., & Seidel, J.V. (1982). Patterns of depression in chronic illness. *Psychotherapy. Psychosomatic, 37*, 144-153.

Coyne, J.C. & Smith, D.A. (1991). Couples coping with a myocardial infarction: A contextual perspective on wives' distress. *Journal of Personality and Social Psychology, 61*, 404-412.

Devins, G.M., Bezjak, A., Mah, K., Loblaw, D.A., & Gotowiec, A.P. (2006). Context moderates illness-induced lifestyle disruptions across life domains: a test of the illness intrusiveness theoretical framework in six common cancers. *Psycho-Oncology. 15*, 221-233.

Devins, G.M., Dion, R., Pelletier, L. G., Shapiro, C.M., Abbey, S., Raiz, L.R., Binik, Y.M., McGowan, P., Kutner, N.G., Beanlands, H., & Edworthy, S.M.(2001). Structure of lifestyle disruptions in chronic disease. *Medical Care, 39*(10), 1097-1104.

Devins, G.M., Binik, Y.M., Hutchinson, T.A., Hollomby, D.J., Barre, P.E. & Guttmann, R.D. (1983). The emotional impact of end-stage renal disease: importance of patients' perceptions of intrusiveness and control. *International Journal of Psychiatry in Medicine, 13(4)*, 327-343.

Diagnostic and Statistical Manual of Mental Disorders, ed 4, TR, Washington DC, American Psychiatric Association, 2000, pp 583-590.

Druley, J.A., & Townsend, A.L. (1998). Self-esteem as a mediator between spousal support and depressive symptoms: a comparison of healthy individuals and individuals coping with arthritis. *Health Psychology, 17*(3), 255-261.

Erkolahti, R.K., Ilonen, T., & Saarijarvi, S. (2003). Self-image of adolescents with diabetes mellitus type-I and rheumatoid arthritis. *Nord J Psychiatry, 57,* 309-312.

Eysenk, H.J. (1975). *Know your own personality.* New York, Penguin Books.

Foote, A.W., Piazza, D., Holcombe, J., Paul, P. & Daffin, P. (1990). Hope self-esteem and social support in persons with multiple sclerosis. *Journal of Neuroscience Nursing, 22,* 155-159.

Fornari, V., Dancyger, I., La Monaca, G., Budman, C., Goodman, B., Kabo, L., & Katz, J. (2001). Can steroid use be a precipitant in the development of an eating disorder? *International Journal of Eating Disorders, 29*(3), 358-362.

Gale, L., Bennett, P.D., Tallon, D., Brooks, E., Munnoch, K., Scheiber-Kounine, C., Fower, C., Sammon, A., Rayter, Z., Farndon, J., & Vedhara, K. (2001). Quality of partner relationship and emotional responses to a health threat. *Health & Medicine, 6*(4), 373-386.

Gregory, S. (2005). Living with chronic illness in the family setting. *Sociology of Health & Illness, 27*(3), 372-392.

Hagborg, W.J.(1993). The Rosenberg Self-Esteem Scale and Harter's Self-Perception Profile for adolescents: A concurrent validity study. *Psychology in Schools, 30,* 132-136.

Hatchett, L., Friend, R., Symister, P. & Wadhwa, N. (1997). Interpersonal expectations, social support, and adjustment to chronic illness. *Journal of Personality and Social Psychology, 73*(3), 560- 573.

Hesselink, A.E., Penninx, B.W.J.H., Schlosser, M.A.G., Wijnhoven, H.A.H., van der Windt, D.A.W.M., Kriegsman, D.M.W., & van Eijk, J. Th. M. (2004). The role of coping resources and coping style in quality of life of patients with asthma or COPD. *Quality of Life Research, 13,* 509-518.

Huurre, T.M., & Aro, H.M.(2002). Long-term psychological effects of persistent chronic illness. A follow- up study of Finnish adolescents aged 16 to 32 years. *European Child and Adolescent Psychiatry, 11,* 85-91.

Ireys, H.T., Gross, S.S., Werthamer-Larsson, L.A., & Kolodner, K.B.(1994). Self-esteem of young adults with chronic health conditions: appraising the effects of perceived impact. *Developmental and Behavioral Pediatrics, 15*(6), 409-415.

Jackson, P.B. (1992). Specifying the buffering hypothesis: Support, strain, and depression. *Social Psychology Quarterly, 55(4),* 363-378.

Jacobson, A.M., Hauser, S.T., Powers, S. & Noam, G. (1984). The influences of chronic illness and ego development on self-esteem in diabetic and psychiatric adolescent patients. *Journal of Youth and Adolescence, 13*(6), 489-507.

Kalibjian, C. (2003). *Straight from the gut: Living with Crohn's disease and Ulcerative Colitis.* O'Reilly. Sebastopol, CA.

Keenan, P.A., & Kuhn, T.W. (1999). Do glucocorticoids have adverse effects on brain function?. *CNS Drugs, 11*(4), 245-251.

Kellerman, J., Zelter, L., Ellenberg, L., Dash, J. & Rigler, D. (1980). Psychological effects of illness in adolescence: anxiety, self-esteem, and perceptions of control. *Journal of Pediatrics, 104,* 126-131.

Kelly, P. C., Cohen, M. L., Walker, W.O., Caskey, O.L., & Atkinson, A.W. (1989). Self-esteem in children medically managed for attention deficit disorder. *Pediatrics, 83*(2), 211-217.

Litt, I.F., Cuskey, W.R., Rosenberg, A. (1982) Role of self-esteem and autonomy in determining medication compliance among adolescents with juvenile rheumatoid arthritis. *Pediatrics, 69*(1), 15-17.

Livneh, H & Antonak, R.F. (2005). Psychosocial adaptation to chronic illness and disability: a primer for counselors. *Journal of Counseling and Development. 83,* 12-20.

Main, J., Moss-Morris, R., Booth, R., Kaptein, A., & Kolbe, J. (2003) The use of reliever medication in asthma: the role of negative mood and symptom reports. *Journal of Asthma. 40*(4), 357-365.

Martinez, S.M., Kemper, C. A., Diamond, C., Wagner, G., & California Collaborative Treatment Group(2005). Body image in patients with HIV/AIDS: assessment of a new psychometric measure and its medical correlates. *AIDS Patient Care and STDs. 19*(3), 150-156.

McCabe, M.P. & Di Battista, J. (2004) Role of health, relationships, work and coping on adjustment among people with multiple sclerosis: A longitudinal investigation. *Psychology, Health, and Medicine. 9*(4), 431-439.

McPherson, K., Steel, C.M. & Dixon, J.M. (2000). Breast cancer-epidemiology, risk factors and genetics. *British Medical Journal, 321,* 624-628.

Meijer, S., Sinnema, G., Bijstra, J., Mellenbergh, G., & Wolters, W. (2000). Social functioning in children with a chronic illness. *Journal of Child Psychology and Psychiatry, 41*(3), 309-317.

Miller, R.C. & Lefcourt, H.M. (1982). The assessment of social intimacy. *Journal of Personality Assessment. 46*(5), 514-518.

Mishel, M.H., & Braden, C.J. (1988). Finding meaning: Antecedents of uncertainty in illness. *Nursing Research, 37,* 98-127.

Mullins, L.L., Cote, M. P., Fuemmeler, B.F., Jean, V.M., Beatty, W.W., & Paul, R.H. (2001). Illness Intrusiveness, uncertainty, and distress in individuals with multiple sclerosis. *Rehabilitation Psychology. 46*(2), 139-153.

Naude, H. & Pretorius, E. (2003). Investigating the effects of asthma medication on the cognitive and psychosocial functioning of primary school children with asthma. *Early Child Development and Care. 173*(6), 699-709.

Nicolson, P. & Anderson, P. (2003) Quality of life, distress and self-esteem: a focus group study of people with chronic bronchitis. *British Journal of Health Psychology, 8*, 251-270.

Norton, T.R., Manne, S.L., Hernandez, E., Rubin, S., Carlson, J., Bergman, C., & Rosenblum, N. (2005). Ovarian cancer patients' psychological distress: the role of physical impairment, perceived unsupported family and friend behaviors, perceived control, and self-esteem. *Health Psychology, 24*(2), 143-152.

Reynolds, W.M. (1982). Development of reliable and valid short forms of the Marlowe-Crowe Social Desirability Scale. *Journal of Clinical Psychology, 38*, 119-125.

Robins, R.W., Hendin, H.M., & Trzesniewski, K.H. (2001).Measuring global self-Esteem: Construct validation of a single-item measure and the Rosenberg Self-Esteem Scale. *Personality and Social Psychology Bulletin, 27(2)*, 151-161.

Rosenberg, M. (1989). *Society and the Adolescent Self-Image.* Revised edition. Middletown, CT, Wesleyan University Press.

Rubin, S.C., Hoskins, W.J., Saigo, P.E., Chapman, D., Hakes, T.B., Markman, M., et al. (1991). Prognostic factors for recurrence following negative second-look Laparotomy in ovarian cancer patients treated with platinum-based chemotherapy. *Gynecologic Oncology, 42,* 137-141.

Scherman, M.H., Dahlgren, L.O. & Lowhagen, O. (2002). Refusing to be ill: a longitudinal study of patients' experiences of asthma/allergy. *Disability and Rehabilitation, 24*(6), 297-307.

Schmidt, S., Petersen, C., & Bullinger, M. (2003). Coping with chronic disease from the perspective of children and adolescents- a conceptual framework and its implications for participation. *Child: Care, Health & Development, 29*(1) 63-75.

Skerrett, K. (2003). Couple dialogues with illness: expanding the "we". *Families, Systems, & Health, 21*(1), 69-80.

Sklar, J. (2002). *A patient-expert walks you through everything you need to learn and do the first year Crohn's Disease and ulcerative colitis.* New York: Marlowe & company.

Silver, E.J., Bauman, L.J., & Ireys, H.T. (1995) Relationships of self-esteem and efficacy psychological distress in mothers of children with chronic physical illnesses. *Health Psychology, 14*(4), 333-340.

Suurmeijer, T.P.B.M., Reuvekamp, M.F., & Aldenkamp, B.P. (2001). Social functioning, psychological functioning, and quality of life in epilepsy. *Epilepsia. 42*(9). 1160-1168.

Symister, P. & Friend, R. (2003). The influence of social support and problematic support on optimism and depression in chronic illness: a prospective study evaluating self-esteem as a mediator. *Health Psychology. 22*(2), 123-129.

van Lankveld, W., Naring, G., van't Pad Bosch, P., & van de Putte. (2000). The negative effect of decreasing the level of activity in coping with pain in rheumatoid arthritis: an increase in psychological distress and disease impact. *Journal of Behavioral Medicine. 23*(4), 377-391.

Walsh, P.A. & Walsh, A. (1987). Self-esteem and disease adaptation among multiple sclerosis patients. *The Journal of Social Psychology, 127*(6), 669-671.

Whiteside-Mansell, L & Corwyn, R.F. (2003). Mean and covariance structures analyses: An examination of the Rosenberg self-esteem scale among adolescents and adults. *Educational and Psychological Measurements. 63,* 163-173.

World Almanac & Book of Facts (2003). Drugs most frequently prescribed in physicians' offices, 2000, 85.

Appendix A

Informed Consent Form

I am informed that this study involves research which will be conducted by Kristin Plachetka M.A., a student at the California School of Professional Psychology, Los Angeles (CSPP-LA) at Alliant International University. I understand that this project is designed to study self-esteem and social intimacy in patients who have taken prednisone. I have been asked to participate in this study because I have taken prednisone for at least three months. If I have not taking prednisone, than I will be used as a comparison group. I understand that my participation in this study will involve the completion of four instruments designed to measure self-esteem, social intimacy and illness intrusion. I am aware that my involvement in this study will take approximately 15 minutes of my time.

I understand that I may refuse to participate or withdraw from this study at any time without any penalty or loss of services that I am entitled to. I understand that my identity as a participant in this study will be kept in strict confidence and that no information that identifies me in any way will be released without my separate written approval. I am aware that all information that identifies me will be protected to the limits allowed by the law.

I have been informed that only Kristin Plachetka and Tracy Heller Ph.D. will have access to data that identifies me personally. I have been informed that all data collected from or about me will be destroyed by Kristin Plachetka within five years of the signing of this document.

I have been informed that some questions in this study may make me feel uncomfortable. I have been informed that the study poses minimal risk of discomfort at introspection that may occur while completing the questionnaires. If this occurs, then Kristin Plachetka, the principal investigator of this project, may be contacted, and, if necessary, a referral will be made for further psychological help at my own expense.

I am aware that although I may not directly benefit from this study, my participation in this project will benefit the field of psychology and medicine.

I understand that I may contact Kristin Plachetka, kplachetka@alliant.edu or her supervisor Tracy Heller Ph.D. CSPP-LA at Alliant International University, 1000 South Fremont Ave. Unit 5, Alhambra, CA 91803 and (626)284-2777 ext. 3049 if I have any questions about this project or my participation in this study. I understand that at the end of the study I may request a summary of results or additional information about the study from Kristin Plachetka.

Please check one of the following options:
_____ I request a summary of the results of this study when it is completed. I may be contacted at the following address to receive a summary of the results:

___ I am not interested in receiving a summary of the results of this study.

I understand that I will be signing two copies of this form. I will keep one copy and Kristin Plachetka will keep the second copy for her records.
I have read this form and I understand what it says. I am 18 years or older and voluntarily agree to participate in this research project.

Participant's Signature	Date

Researcher's Signature	Date

Appendix B

Rosenberg Self-Esteem Scale

This scale may be obtained from:

The Morris Rosenberg Foundation
c/o Dept. of Sociology
University of Maryland
2112 Art/Soc Building
College Park, MD 20742-1315

Appendix C

Miller Social Intimacy Scale

This scale may be obtained from:

Dr. Rickey Miller
Toronto General Hospital
Eaton N 8-238
101 College St.
Toronto, Ont., Canada M5G167

Appendix D

Adapted Illness Intrusiveness Ratings

This scale may be obtained from:

Stanford Patient Education Research Center
1000 Welch Road., Suite 204
Palo Alto, CA 94304

Appendix E

Demographics

Please answer each question or check the appropriate answer.

1. Gender
   ___ Male
   ___ Female

2. Age: _____

3. Ethnicity
   ___ Caucasian
   ___ Latino
   ___ African-American
   ___ Asian-American/ Pacific Islander
   ___ Multi-Ethnic _____
   ___ Other _____

4. Marital Status, check all that apply
   ___ Single, not dating
   ___ Single, dating
   ___ Married
   ___ Committed relationship
   ___ Divorced
   ___ Widowed

5. Education
   ___ some high school
   ___ high school graduate
   ___ some college
   ___ college graduate
   ___ some graduate school
   ___ graduate school degree(example Ph. D., Ed, MD)

6. Approximate annual income: _____

7. Employment status
   ___ Student
   ___ Part-time employment
   ___ Full-time employment
   ___ Unemployed
   ___ Disability

8. Have you been diagnosed with a chronic illness? ____ yes or ____ no

9. What chronic illness have you been diagnosed with?
   ____ asthma
   ____ Crohn's disease or Ulcerative colitis
   ____ Rheumoid arthritis
   ____ diabetes
   ____ cancer
   ____ HIV/AIDS
   ____ Multiple Sclerosis
   ____ heart disease
   ____ other _____

10. How long ago were you diagnosed with a chronic illness?
    ____ months   or ____ years

11. At what age were you diagnosed with a chronic illness? ____ years

12. Are you currently on any medication? ____ yes or ____ no

13. Have you ever taken a medication for three months or more? ____ yes or ____ no

14. At what age were you first given a medication for a chronic illness? ____ years

15. What medication(s) are you currently taking?
    ____ Remicade
    ____ Humira
    ____ Prednisone
    ____ insulin
    ____ Methotrexate
    ____ Lipitor
    ____ Albuterol
    ____ Other(please list) _____

16. What medication(s) have you taken in the past?
    ____ Remicade, if so for how long?_____
    ____ Humira, if so for how long?_____
    ____ Prednisone, if so for how long?_____
    ____ insulin, if so for how long?_____
    ____ Methotrexate, if so for how long?_____
    ____ Lipitor, if so for how long?_____
    ____ Albuterol, if so for how long?_____
    ____ Other(please list) if so for how long?_____

    _____

17. If you are not currently taking medication, how long ago did you last take medication for treatment of a chronic illness?
    ___ months ago or ____ years ago

18. Have you ever taken prednisone?   ____ yes or ____ no

19. Have you ever taken prednisone for three months or more?   ____ yes or ____ no

20. Are you currently taking prednisone?   ____ yes or ____ no

21. If you are currently taking prednisone, how long have you been taking prednisone?
    ____ months or ____ years

22. If you are not currently taking prednisone, when was your last dose of prednisone?
    _____ months ago or ____ years ago

23. Have you ever taken 10mg or more of prednisone a day?   ____ yes or ____ no

24. Are you currently experiencing any side effects from a medication used in the treatment of a chronic illness?   ____ yes or ____ no

25. If yes, which side effects are you CURRENTLY experiencing from a medication for a chronic illness? (Check all that apply) And circle the severity of the side effect experienced. Please fill out side effects questions about the medication(s) you have taken most recently.

	None	Mild	Moderate		Severe	
Rounding of the Face	0	1	2	3	4	5
Stretch Marks	0	1	2	3	4	5
Weight Gain	0	1	2	3	4	5
Hair Loss	0	1	2	3	4	5
Increased Facial Hair Growth	0	1	2	3	4	5
Mood Swings	0	1	2	3	4	5
Acne	0	1	2	3	4	5
Unusual Tiredness	0	1	2	3	4	5
Nausea	0	1	2	3	4	5
Difficulty Sleeping	0	1	2	3	4	5
Dry Mouth	0	1	2	3	4	5
Headache	0	1	2	3	4	5
Sexual Side Effects	0	1	2	3	4	5
Dizziness	0	1	2	3	4	5
Other _____	0	1	2	3	4	5

26. What medications caused these side effects?

_____

27. Which side effects are you bothered by the most?

_____

28. How much do medication side effects interfere with your personal relationships? (circle the choice that best matched the level of interference)

None	A little		Somewhat		Very Much
0	1	2	3	4	5

29. How much do medication side effects interfere with your self-esteem? (circle the choice that best matched the level of interference)

None	A little		Somewhat		Very Much
0	1	2	3	4	5

27. How much are you bothered by medication side effects? Please circle the appropriate answer.

	None	Mildly		Moderately	Severely	
Rounding of the Face	0	1	2	3	4	5
Stretch Marks	0	1	2	3	4	5
Weight Gain	0	1	2	3	4	5
Hair Loss	0	1	2	3	4	5
Increased Facial Hair Growth	0	1	2	3	4	5
Mood Swings	0	1	2	3	4	5
Acne	0	1	2	3	4	5
Unusual Tiredness	0	1	2	3	4	5
Nausea	0	1	2	3	4	5
Difficulty Sleeping	0	1	2	3	4	5
Dry Mouth	0	1	2	3	4	5
Headache	0	1	2	3	4	5
Sexual Side Effects	0	1	2	3	4	5
Dizziness	0	1	2	3	4	5
Other _____	0	1	2	3	4	5

CPSIA information can be obtained at www.ICGtesting.com
Printed in the USA
BVOW07s1412310314

349299BV00008B/543/P